DRIVE, EGO, OBJECT, AND SELF

DRIVE, EGO, OBJECT, AND SELF

A Synthesis for Clinical Work

FRED PINE

BasicBooks
A Division of HarperCollins*Publishers*

Excerpts from: Bornstein, B. (1949). The analysis of a phobic child. *Psychoanalytic Study of the Child*, 3/4, 181–226. Reprinted with permission of International Universities Press, Inc.

Excerpts from: Fleming, J. (1975). Some observations on object constancy in the psychoanalysis of adults. *Journal of the American Psychoanalytic Association*, 23, 743–759. Reprinted with permission of International Universities Press, Inc.

Excerpts from: Loewald, H. W. (1971). On motivation and instinct theory. *Psychoanalytic Study of the Child*, 26. Copyright © 1972 by Ruth S. Eissler, Anna Freud, Marianne Kris, and Seymour L. Lustman. Reprinted by permission of Yale University Press.

Excerpts from: Mitchell, S. A. (1984). Object relations theories and the developmental tilt. *Contemporary Psychoanalysis*, 20, 473–499. Reprinted with permission.

Excerpts from: Pine, F. (1985). *Developmental theory and clinical process*. Copyright © 1985 by Yale University. Reprinted by permission of Yale University Press.

Excerpts from: Pine F. (1986a). On the development of the "borderline-child-to-be." *American Journal of Orthopsychiatry*, 56, 450–457. Copyright © 1986 by the *American Journal of Orthopsychiatry*. Reprinted with permission.

Excerpts from: Pine, F. (1986b). The "symbiotic phase" in the light of current infancy research. *Bulletin of the Menninger Clinic*, 50, 564–569. Reprinted with permission.

Excerpts from: Pine, F. (1988). The four psychologies of psychoanalysis and their place in clinical work. *Journal of the American Psychoanalytic Association*, 36, 571–596. Reprinted with permission of International Universities Press, Inc.

Excerpts from: Pine, F. (1989). Motivation, personality organization, and the four psychologies of psychoanalysis. *Journal of the American Psychoanalytic Association*, 37, 27–60. Reprinted with permission of International Universities Press, Inc.

Excerpts from: Segel, N. P. (1981). Narcissism and adaptation to indignity. *International Journal of Psychoanalysis*, 62, 465–476. Copyright © Institute of Psycho-Analysis. Reprinted with permission.

Library of Congress Cataloging-in-Publication Data
Pine, Fred, 1931–
    Drive, ego, object, and self : a synthesis for clinical work /
Fred Pine.
      p.   cm.
    Includes bibliographical references (p.).
    ISBN 0–465–01722–3
    1. Psychoanalysis.   I. Title.
    RC504.P56   1990
    616.89'17—dc20   89–43168
                                         CIP

To Rachael and Daniel

Contents

Preface

THE PHENOMENA OF clinical work, as they are conceptualized today, are often seen as falling into four broad domains. We are accustomed to referring to these domains as those of drive, ego, object relations, and self. Our theories ought to fit with these observations and to suggest how things got that way. My aim in this book is to propose a view along those lines.

Whatever original contribution there is herein, it is not intended to be in the groupings of the phenomena themselves, nor in the broad conceptual languages used to describe them. There I shall simply work with our familiar terms: drive, ego, object relations, self. I recognize that these are loose and overlapping groupings, and that the phenomena could be grouped in other ways; but they are familiar, and I am used to rediscovering them continually in clinical work, and so I shall stay with them here. I wish to emphasize at the outset that I will be focusing on the *phenomena*, not formal theories regarding them—thus self, but not Self Psychology; object relations, but not the views of any one theorist; and drive and ego, but not only in the ways they have been addressed in classical psychoanalysis.

As phenomena, they have been part of the data of observation ever since the way of thinking that we call psychoanalysis came into being in Freud's writings. Certainly drive concepts were central in his work—in his varying dual instinct theories and in the continuing centrality he accorded to sexuality, broadly conceived. An ego concept was present from the start, alternately referred to under the broad heading of "defense" or the narrower one of "repression." This is certainly familiar. But object relations and self were also important in Freud's writings. He gave recognition to the significance of the object in couching the stages of core anxiety in the language of separation—loss of the object, and loss of the love of the object, his first two stages, most notably; and transference and the oedipal constellation are as much object relations concepts as they are drive concepts. As for self, though he put it in quasi-libidinal/instinctual terms, Freud's struggles with the concept of narcissism were efforts to deal with the experience of "self," the person's relation to the self as object. It seems that drive, ego, object relations, and self *are* the phenomena of mental life, or are at least central among them, and we rediscover them again and again.

My own contribution is intended to be in the attempt at some synthesis of these phenomena (actually a clinical demonstration that they *are* synthesized in individual persons) and a developmental argument regarding how they got that way. Since in itself this is, I recognize, an ambitious attempt, I hasten to add what the views to be presented do not attempt to do. They do not represent a formal theory; there is no metatheory here, no basic postulates that serve as firm anchor points. Rather, I step into the developmental and clinical processes in midstream and try to make some sense of them. And I skirt the issue of hermeneutics versus science that is currently actively argued in the psychoanalytic literature, recognizing that my arguments can be drawn into either position.

My own statement is offered in three main parts: a theoretical section where the point of view is developed; a clinical section where it is illustrated; and an applied section where I utilize the ideas, along with further clinical examples, to attempt some clarification of various current issues in the psychoanalytic literature.

Among the broad set of ideas presented here, I introduced some in my earlier book, *Developmental Theory and Clinical Process* (1985); but I rapidly came to the opinion that that was only an introduction—that there was a lot more to be said about them. Hence the fuller statement with clinical illustrations in the present book.

Acknowledgments

I WANT TO express my gratitude, first, to the individuals who worked with me in their personal psychoanalyses and who gave me permission to describe aspects of those analyses here. From the start I felt that the book would require extensive illustrative clinical reports. This led to a long delay in the writing, however, as I was naturally hesitant to publish such private material. Eventually I decided to proceed in a way that felt professionally sound, and this included (in addition, of course, to appropriate disguise) seeking the permission of the patients whose clinical material was to appear in the book. What I did was the following: I first worked on the manuscript and the case reports until they reached their final form; only then did I seek permission (so that I was in a position to show the write-ups to patients in that final form); and only after that did I conclude that I could go ahead and publish. This final product is the outcome of that process, and I again express my gratitude to the individuals who allowed me the use of the material described herein.

The process of requesting permissions itself turned out to be both educative and moving, sometimes profoundly so, for both the analysands (past and current) and me. They read the write-ups, commented on them, and sometimes recommended changes or additions—all of which are reflected in the final presentations here. But more significantly, the whole process—the approach by me as well as the reading of the contents of the write-ups—stimulated analytic work in various ways. With individuals currently in analysis, of course, it became part of the analytic work; and I have no doubt that it will continue to be a presence in that work throughout the analyses. With individuals who had completed their analyses, and whom I recontacted to seek permission, it stimulated a reworking and reevaluation of both their analysis and their relationship to me.

Since the issue is such a problematic one for psychoanalytic writing, I want to say that the process to date seems to have been not destructive but rather productive as it is itself subjected to analytic work or postanalytic review. I am not so naive as to think that this particular "parameter" is ever fully "analyzed away," but in that, I believe it joins much else in an analysis of which that same can be said (and often with respect to things of which the analyst is not even aware). But certainly, in the present instance, real work has gone on in relation to this new fact in the analysis, and I expect that to continue. Nonetheless, I cannot say how things will work out over the long term and whether untoward complications may develop. I respectfully hope that no seriously problematic issues arise.

Second, I wish to thank a few individuals who have been extremely helpful in enabling me to get this book written. Dr. Herman van Praag, Chairman of the Department of Psychiatry at the Albert Einstein College of Medicine, met my request for a sabbatical cooperatively, and it was during that sabbatical in the second half of 1987 that the first draft of this work got written. I am pleased to express my thanks to him.

Ms. Marie Mele, my secretary at the College of Medicine and an extraordinarily competent person, made that competence available to me as she produced beautiful working and final drafts of the manuscript. That she did this while working under my self-imposed time pressure (which I regularly placed right on her desk along with the manuscript) only increases my gratitude.

Jo Ann Miller, Director of Professional Books at Basic Books, could always be counted upon for clear and straight-thinking commentary, in relation to this book and in my previous contacts with her; I value that highly. Her assistant, Andrea Ben-Yosef, has been helpful at every turn. And I appreciate the work done by Nola Lynch, who copyedited this book.

Finally, I wish to acknowledge those editors and publishers who granted permission for me to incorporate material that I had published elsewhere, often in quite different forms from their appearance herein. Formal acknowledgment is given on the copyright page, but I wish to describe the present use of those works. I draw upon two papers that first appeared in the *Journal of the American Psychoanalytic Association* (Pine, 1988, 1989), using them here in revised and extended form. The first of these appears in this book as part of chapters 2, 3, and 12; the second appears here, with modifications and extensions, as part of chapters 5 and 6. Portions of two other prepublished papers are also drawn upon in this book. A small section of chapter 10, on the development of specific ego capacities, first appeared in the *American Journal of Orthopsychiatry* (Pine, 1986a) as part of a larger, quite different paper. And what appears here as chapter 11, is a substantially enlarged and altered version of a paper that first appeared in the *Bulletin of the Menninger Clinic* (Pine, 1986b). And last, a brief historically oriented literature review that appears here as part of chapter 2 was published in similar form by Yale University Press in my previous book (Pine, 1985). Permissions to utilize extensive quotations from other authors are also indicated on the copyright page. I am grateful for each of these permissions to republish.

Although all of the case studies in this book are real, the names and identifying details of the individuals mentioned have been changed in order to protect their privacy.

DRIVE, EGO, OBJECT, AND SELF

PART I

THEORETICAL

IN THIS PART, I present a clinically and developmentally based model that moves toward an integration of the four major current psychoanalytic psychologies—those of drive, ego, object relations, and self. The ideas presented represent a coalescence of two modes of thinking. One mode begins with what we see clinically and asks, how could this have come about developmentally? The other, in reverse, begins with the observational domain of infant and child development and asks: what are the likely later clinical manifestations of the observed phenomena? what are their intrapsychic components? and which of these become most central, and how? The answers to these questions are guided by knowledge of outcomes that are actually seen clinically later on.

In seeking to account for how clinical phenomena come to include aspects of drive, ego, object relations, and self—each potentially as a central organization—I look closely at individual development. And there I believe we find that no one of the four has developmental priority; each of the four

1

has very early origins and a long course of development. My main point is that they become increasingly interrelated with one another, that each of the four achieves motivational status and thus can become a dynamically central organization—entering into the causal chain of behavior.

The overall view of human psychological functioning that underlies and results from the concepts to be developed here is consistent with the psychoanalytic emphasis on the centrality of *conflict*. But it will give equal centrality to the place of *repetition* and of *development*, the latter referring to both normal and blocked or aberrant development.

Clinical illustrations are reserved for the second and third parts of the book.

CHAPTER 1

Multiple Perspectives and Singular Persons

OVER THE DECADES, psychoanalysts have evolved a number of perspectives on intrapsychic life to help make sense of the data of clinical psychoanalysis. Each takes a somewhat different view of human functioning, emphasizing somewhat different phenomena. I shall refer to those perspectives that are central currently as the four psychologies of psychoanalysis—the psychologies of drive, ego, object relations, and self experience. By calling them psychologies, I mean to emphasize the claim each makes to describing a significant way in which the mind functions. And by calling them psychologies of psychoanalysis, I mean to emphasize that each lays claim also to a complex, in-depth view of the mind based on the shaping influence of early bodily based and object-connected experiences. Each of them adds something new to our understanding.

Each of the four conceptual domains, while having a certain degree of internal consistency, is also to a degree only a loose grouping of phenomena. And certainly at the edges, so to speak, they overlap with one another.

Phenomena are continuous, not categorical—especially in a site as complex as the human mind. And so, even with attention to a set of four clinically relevant domains of phenomena, the conceptual fit to the actualities of clinical work remains imperfect.

To the degree that individual theorists and clinicians are excessively ardent in their support of one or another of these psychologies, I believe they are in the familiar position of the blind men and the elephant, each touching a different part and mistaking the part for the whole animal. The complexity of the human animal is sufficiently great such that we gain in our understanding by having multiple perspectives upon it. The perspectives on the elephant vary spatially; the view you get depends on where you touch—legs, tail, tusks, or trunk. But the perspectives on human functioning, I shall argue, vary temporally. We all function differently and are intrapsychically organized differently at different moments. The view you get depends on when you are looking.

But though our potential perspectives are multiple, the persons they refer to are nonetheless singular—in both senses of the term. They are one (whole, integrated), though with plenty of room for conflict (and it shall be one of my tasks to propose modes of integration of the diversity). And persons are singular in the sense of unique, each different from the other (and the multiple perspectives better provide the tools for describing the full array of that uniqueness).

While I shall develop an integrated view of the several perspectives provided by the four psychologies, I shall not be making any effort to integrate general theories or the views of particular theorists. That task is too cumbersome, probably not possible to do, and in any event quite aside from my intent. My intent instead is to work toward an integrative view of the substantive phenomena to which the various theories address themselves: phenomena such as urges (in the drive psychology); modes of defense and adaptation (in the ego psychology); relationships and their internalization, distortion, and repetition (in the object relations psychology); and phenomena of differentiation and boundary formation, of personal agency and authenticity, and of self-esteem (in the self psychology). In not granting any automatic primacy to drive theory, I do not mean to reject the centrality—indeed the all-pervasiveness—of conflict. Quite the reverse. By recognizing and respecting the multiplicity of variables central to human function that have been highlighted by diverse theorists I hope to increase the space in our theories for complexity—complexity reflected in the central place of conflict and of the multiple functions of behavior.

This wide-ranging integrative attempt is an outgrowth of clinical experience and developmental study. It seems to me to fit, or at least reasonably approximate, the realities of those two domains. As for the clinical domain, a look at the major psychoanalytic journals makes clear that clinical work has expanded in recent years with regard to patient populations worked with, clinical phenomena seen, theories used to organize these phenomena, and interpretive approaches used within an analysis. My aim in this book is to advance a view of motivation and personality organization that could be seen to underlie, be implicit in, or provide a framework for this expansion. A multiperspective approach, I believe, underlies the way many analysts in fact work with their patients today. And as for the developmental domain, the view of the person accorded by infant and child observation is very different from the view accorded by the clinical psychoanalytic looking glass. If in clinical psychoanalysis persistent wishes can be seen as central organizers of the in-session associative material, in infant and child observation relationships and their distortions, adaptations and their failure, and the dawning awareness of a self, an "I," press themselves upon virtually all observers. Our theories should aspire to reflect this full range of phenomena.

Let me begin with two brief sets of illustrations: a hypothetical clinical example and a developmental example.

A HYPOTHETICAL CLINICAL EXAMPLE

Let us imagine a not uncommon clinical history—a woman who had had, as a child, a flirtatious sexualized relation to her father of a degree that was intensely exciting to her and who suffered a profound sense of rebuff when she felt she lost him when her mother was near. In the session to be imagined, she was flirtatious with her male analyst. Other imagined session content will be assumed to vary, according to the point I wish to make and will be referred to in the hypothetical interpretations.

Interpretations to such a patient would be responsive to the in-session content, of course, and would be based upon how her central motivations were understood—which motive(s) seemed active at this particular time in this particular session. Thus, depending on general clinical circumstances and the specific session content, one can envision any of the following as an appropriate interpretation:

1. So, now that your mother has left for her vacation, you seem to feel safe in being flirtatious here, too, as you say you've been all day with others. I guess you're figuring that this time, finally, I won't turn away to be with her as you felt your father did.
2. It's not surprising that you suddenly found yourself retelling that incident of the time when your mother was critical of you. I think you were critical of yourself for flirting with me so freely just now, and you brought her right into the room with us so that nothing more could happen between us.
3. Your hope seems to be that, if you continue to get excitedly flirtatious with me, and I don't respond with excitement, you'll finally be able to tolerate your excitement without fearing that you'll be overwhelmed by it.
4. When those profound feelings of emptiness arise in you, the flirtatiousness helps you feel filled and alive, and so it becomes especially precious to you. It was as though, when your father turned his attention to your mother, he didn't know that you had wished to be healed by him and not only sexy with him.

These are invented interpretations for an invented session. I hope it is obvious that what is actually said by the analyst in a session would be based on what actually is said by the patient in that session and on the transference situation as it is then manifest. In that context, the interpretation offered (from among an infinite range of possibilities) would be tailored to how this particular material in this particular patient in this particular session seemed best understood. No analyst, we hope, would bring to a session a theory-dictated, preformed interpretation.

But my point is that the range of interpretations actually used by analysts draws on widely varying "contents" of human history or "processes" of human functioning. Thus, the first "interpretation" given is meant to highlight the effort to gratify a sexually powered wish in a relatively uncomplicated fashion. The second interpretation centers on guilt and defense; it draws on the ideas that the flirtation aroused anxiety and guilt and that the memory of the object relationship to the mother could be used for defensive purposes—both to express and externalize the blame-saying (mother criticizes her, not she herself) and to defend against the flirtatious intimacy (mother is made to be present in thought). The third interpretation focuses on repetition in efforts after mastery; it draws on the idea that even supposedly pleasurable affect in object-relational experiences can reach traumatic (unmasterable) levels of intensity that produce repetitive efforts to master the still-blocked psychic tension. And the fourth interpretation centers on a painful subjective experience of self; it draws on the idea that erotic arousal (or any strong affect) can itself be used defensively to ward off intolerable feelings of emptiness or depression. Though each of these interpretations have been tailored, for purposes of explication here, to highlight different aspects of psychological function—sexual gratification, defense, repetition of an old object relationship, and self experience—no one of these views of human function is the exclusive possession of any one formal psychological theory. They are all aspects of human function and of necessity are addressed by all serious and encompassing theories.

I have given four hypothetical interpretations to introduce an aspect of my theme. But they are hypothetical only in the sense that they are based on a fictitious instance and a session that did not in fact happen. They certainly are within the range of the kinds of interpretation that I find myself drawing on regularly in day-to-day work. In that sense, they are not at all hypothetical. And, in principle, at different times, each of these interpretations and more might be given to the same patient, as the analysis revealed different aspects of the "same" event.

I suspect that such a range of interpretation is part of the work of most clinical psychoanalysts. But explicitly espoused theories do not always reflect this full range. The relation between theory and clinical practice, altogether, is very difficult to describe for something as complex, ever varying, and nonreproducible as an analysis. We tend to elevate to the level of theory those particular concepts that are useful to us as primary organizers; and we then espouse different theories. While I am not suggesting that all analysts in fact really *work* alike, I am suggesting that clinical work is often more widely varying than our theories reflect. In psychoanalysis, theories—

though complex—inevitably simplify. I hope to give complexity itself a more central place in theory.

To aim in this direction, as already noted, is not necessarily to aim for an integration of the various *theories* themselves. Freud's (1905) drive theory, Heinz Hartmann's (1939) ego psychology, W.R.D. Fairbairn's (1941) object relations theory, and Heinz Kohut's (1977) Self Psychology—as examples—all carry a lot of metapsychological baggage; and it is not my aim to pull all of that together. But each of the theories does highlight particular aspects of the substantive *phenomena* of human functioning, and I shall endeavor to develop a view which gives place to all of them.

One final point on this introductory clinical example. Just as work with the phenomena of drive, of ego function, of object relations, and of self experience does not require adopting the several metapsychologies that theorists have tied to them, neither does it require working clinically in four (or however many) different ways. My own way of working involves quiet listening, relative anonymity, neutrality, nongratification of drive aims, and interpretation (or question asking). The principal variation in what I propose is in the substantive content of mental life addressed by interpretation, and this depends on how the central and active motives underlying what we see are understood at any particular moment in a particular patient. (I do believe we have to vary our interventions along a "holding environment" axis—see Winnicott, 1963b; Modell, 1984; Pine, 1985—depending on the difficulty of the clinical moment for the patient, but this applies across all four of the psychologies and is merely an extension and elaboration of what usually has gone under the names of clinical tact and timing.)

A DEVELOPMENTAL EXAMPLE

This time let us imagine a not-at-all hypothetical infant; rather, any and all infants. Here the imagining has to do with the effort to feel our way into the infant's subjective experience. But we do this based on our own subjective experiences, and those of already verbal children and adults. The inferences are not drawn simply from thin air. But even if I (and others who think similarly) may be pushing these subjective experiences too far back in time (into the period of infancy), it does not affect the central thrust of the argument I wish to make here: that psychological experience is organized in different ways at different moments, and that these differences in the forms of psychological experience are part of what underlie and provide the basis for the differences in the several psychologies of drive, ego, object relations, and self.

So let us imagine a three-month-old infant, quietly wakeful, looking around at his surroundings, making some gurgling sounds—altogether in a state of what Peter Wolff (1959) has described as "alert inactivity" or what D. W. Winnicott (1956) has described as "going on being" (that is, quietly existing without the experience of disturbing impingements). As time passes, however, an impingement does come. Hunger mounts. With its first mild beginnings, the infant manages to find his thumb. And, thumb in mouth, sucking mildly, he can continue looking around. But hunger mounts further and as it does it increasingly commands attention. The thumb no longer distracts. No longer is the infant quietly gurgling and looking around. Crying begins and the "going-on-being" state is erased. But then the mother, hearing the cries from another room, calls out in a singsong voice, "Hello! I'm coming!" And the infant pauses in his crying and looks toward the door. The mother enters smiling. For several moments the infant smiles responsively. But then hunger and crying take over again, until the mother starts to feed him. At first, there is vigorous sucking, and then the movement toward satiation and quiescence begins. Continuing the sucking, the infant begins to relax, body tonus diminishes, and he melts off into sleep against his mother's body.

What discrete moments, what differing patterns of experience, can we tease out of this scenario? At the outset of the chosen incident, the infant—looking around and gurgling—is unself-consciously engaged in the exercise of his visual and vocal apparatus, and taking in aspects of his surround, his external reality. All of this—exercise of function and appraisal of reality—is addressed by a psychology of ego function. That is, the development of psychologically relevant tools of functioning and the learning and use of the world of reality are among the substantive phenomena addressed by the psychology of what we refer to as ego functioning.

The description of that moment of ego function is based on observation. But now let me draw on inference to turn to a second, possible intrapsychic, moment. The fact that hunger can be described as an impingement

(Winnicott, 1960b) alerts us to ask, an impingement on what? And here I think it is fair to wonder about that quiet, looking around and gurgling, pre-hunger state of the infant—the state upon which hunger impinges. Winnicott (1956) refers to this as a state of "going on being," and we can conjecture about its quality of a not yet self-conscious forerunner of a subjective state of self. A period of *being*, of self experience. Perhaps such a state is phenomenologically highlighted in infant experience by contrasts—that is, by its loss through interruption by hunger. Speculative, yes; but not at all foreign to adult (or even child) experience. Such considerations, and such a state, are central to a psychology of self experience.

And now a third moment can be abstracted from the flow of experience described. Winnicott (1960a) suggests that, early on, biological urges may not yet be experienced as internal by the infant. They are impingements on the ongoing state of being and "can be as much external as a clap of thunder or a hit" (p. 141). And in the instance I selected, as hunger mounts, and, again later, after the moments of delay when the infant finds his thumb or hears his mother's voice, when nursing begins, here we have the beginnings of those psychological experiences central to a psychology of drive—experiences of urge and its tensions, its delays, its satisfactions. Naturally this is just the beginning. Psychic representation of biological urges and their seemingly infinite possibilities for transformation and elaboration has barely begun at this point.

Turn now to the moment when the infant finds his thumb and sucks. Of course this moment of thumbsucking is relevant to a psychology of drive, but I wish to emphasize another aspect of it. When the infant finds his thumb, temporarily reducing the hunger tension and thereby permitting the continuance of gazing, he also demonstrates a piece of what is addressed by a psychology of ego function—here under the broad rubric of defense. In this instance, we do not yet see purely intrapsychic defense; and we may not yet feel comfortable describing this as defense against anxiety. But we have a self-initiated action (thumb to mouth) that serves to modulate the force of a need and, thus, can be broadly conceived as a forerunner to those later intrapsychic (defense) acts that serve to temper urge or reduce anxiety. The defensive use of thumbsucking is even more apparent in the later, established, thumbsucker, whose thumb will go to mouth at any distress—the mother preparing to leave, a parental argument, the child accidentally breaking something, and so on. Here its separateness from hunger is clear, though of course (like some later masturbation) thumbsucking still demonstrates the potential for the person's use of gratification for defensive purposes.

Now one further aspect of the described instance—the moment when the infant, hearing the mother's voice, pauses in his crying, looks toward the door, then smiles responsively when his mother enters smiling. Here we see the evidence for an internally carried (learned) object-relational experience that creates a good inner feeling and permits anticipation of coming satisfaction and hence delay (momentarily) of crying. There is, when the mother calls and enters, an actual engagement with the mother; but there is also, if the call permits delay of crying, evidence of a remembered prior relation that can serve functionally in the present. Such are among the substantive phenomena central to a psychology of object relations.

And finally, in the adduced instance, the moment following sucking—as the infant falls into sleep and melts (with relaxed tonus) into the mother's body—can be seen as another state of self. This time it is a state of "merger," of boundarylessness (see Pine, 1985, 1986b; Mahler, Pine, and Bergman, 1975)—also addressed as an aspect of the psychology of self experience (see chapter 11).

The point I wish to make with both of my examples, clinical and developmental, is that there is a wide range of substantive phenomena in both the clinical and developmental areas that are potentially addressable in ways that I have been subsuming under the term *four psychologies*. And things can go wrong in any of these areas, depending upon the infant's or child's specific vulnerabilities and the specific psychopathology that the primary caretakers bring to the interaction with the child (see chapter 11). These diverse phenomena have been addressed by theorists of different persuasions who have contributed to our understanding of one or another aspect of human development and functioning. It turns out that the diverse ways of understanding phenomena in the clinical situation are matched by parallel ways in developmental observation. Of course, ultimately, there is only one psychology, the one that describes the full range of such development and functioning in all of us. But our understanding has developed piecemeal and, for my purposes here, it will be most useful to continue to refer to a set of four psychologies.

In the child, the diverse sets of phenomena subsumable under concepts of drive, ego, object relations, and self experience can be viewed as differing centers or forms of psychologically significant activity. In this light, our conceptual task and the aim of this book can be seen as the study of the elaboration over time (the question of development) and the integration within the person (the question of psychological structure) of the phenomena of the four psychologies. As I have already indicated, these forms of psychological activity are not absolute and nonoverlapping, of course, and one can see aspects of the others in any single instance of one. But, while for some purposes it is a gain to see the overlap, for others, as I will attempt to show, it is a gain to bear in mind the differences.

In their excellent book surveying the full gamut of psychoanalytic theorists according to their position along an axis varying from a "drive model" (which is more intra-individual) to a "relational model" (more inter-individual), Jay Greenberg and Stephen Mitchell (1983) say that mixing of the two models is inherently unstable because the models are fundamentally incompatible. In illustration of this (see their chapter 11), they review the work of Kohut (1971, 1977) and Joseph Sandler (1976, 1981; Sandler and Rosenblatt, 1962; Sandler and Sandler, 1978), whom they consider "mixed-model" theorists, endeavoring to show that each eventually moved more in one direction and away from the mix. But such an illustration does nothing to advance the idea of a "fundamental incompatibility" (p. 403) between the models; it demonstrates only the direction of development of the thinking of those individuals.

Greenberg and Mitchell argue that, if we are to develop a mixed-model theory, we would need to develop also the "conceptual glue" (p. 352) to hold them together. Clearly, I am working with such a mixed model, perhaps a veritable hodgepodge of models. I will argue that our concepts (of drive, ego, object relations, self) have developed in recognition of the diversity of significant experience. But I will contend that no conceptual glue is needed to hold them together—that is, no glue at the level of a metapsychology that is over and above experience. The way they are held together, that is, the way these diverse phenomena become integrated in any one individual, is itself a product of development and a task of development. There *are* different phenomena, and they *do* become integrated. This is the story of development as I will endeavor to tell it. Our concepts need not provide the glue, but rather give us the terms for describing its natural development.

THE PSYCHOANALYTIC PSYCHOLOGIES:
WHY THESE FOUR?

The questions come up: why four? and why these particular four psychologies: drive, ego, object relations, and self?* Broadly speaking, under these four terms I am referring, respectively, to the domains of (a) drives, urges, wishes; (b) defense, adaptation, reality testing, and defects in the development of each; (c) relationships to significant others *as experienced* and as carried in memory, with whatever attendant distortions such experiences and memories may entail; and (d) subjective experience of self in relation to such phenomena as boundaries, esteem, authenticity, and agency. To go into the four substantively and in any greater detail at this point would feel like a detour; I reserve that discussion for chapter 2. So I shall assume that the reader of this book has enough familiarity with the current psychoanalytic literature that the four terms evoke a broad set of meanings. That general set of meanings will be sufficient backdrop for the particular points I wish to develop here.

Why these four? Is this an exhaustive list? In particular, I have been asked: what of a psychology of superego? or of interpersonal relations? For now, it makes most sense to me to think of superego as a significant part of both the object relations psychology (with respect to identification) and the drive psychology (with particular respect to aggressive drive). And I see interpersonal relations not as a separate psychology, but as one of the domains (the other being the intrapsychic) where the other four are played out. But clearly these are conceptual choices and, though I shall repeatedly emphasize my focus on substantive phenomena, I do not want to overdo the idea of their absolute factuality or independence. I cannot argue that my list is either exhaustive or mutually exclusive; thus, I have also been asked whether I see room for a fifth or a sixth psychology, and whether the list can go on and on. My answer to that is, in principle, yes—if someone comes along and alerts us to new regions of phenomena significant in the psychoanalytic experience and of a sufficient degree of generality. But I do not see that happening soon or often.

These four psychologies all emanate from psychoanalytic listening. They

---

*The writing of this whole section was initiated by questions posed to me by Elizabeth A. Sharpless, Ph.D., after hearing what is now chapter 5 presented at an open lecture. I wish to thank her for those thoughtful questions.

reflect the understandings we develop of intrapsychic life from the viewing points of free association and transference. And from those points of view, they have a good fit with the phenomena we see and work with in psychoanalysis. They have to do with the content of lives, viewed psychoanalytically.

I emphasize the psychoanalytic viewing point bearing in mind an assumption and a caution put forth by Hans Loewald (1971a):

> The psychoanalyst's interpretations are based on and make use of a fundamental assumption: whatever transpires is personally motivated. This assumption is the all embracing interpretation that constitutes the foundation for all individual interpretations. . . . I have implied that the object of psychoanalysis is the individual human person. Only in this entity do we encounter what psychoanalysis calls psychic life and psychic reality. It is the unit with which we deal. This, of course, does not mean that no general statements and propositions can be made about this reality. *But it does mean that psychoanalytic statements and propositions are valid specifically in respect to this entity as conceived in the basic interpretive assumption mentioned and as apprehended in the psychoanalytic method which is determined by this assumption.* Psychoanalytic statements are not necessarily valid in respect to other units, such as for instance family or society, even though these are composed of individuals; nor are they necessarily valid or pertinent for psychological phenomena taken out of the context of the unit constituted by the individual, as is the case in experimental or general psychology. (pp. 103–104) [Emphasis added.]

So when I say that I shall work with the psychologies of drive, ego, object relations, and self because they reflect our understanding of intrapsychic life achieved from the viewing points of free association and transference in the psychoanalytic situation, I am emphasizing both their particularity for and their usefulness *in that situation.* And yet, in this instance, we can follow that "unit," the "individual human person," into at least one other region and find the four psychologies relevant and useful once again. I have in mind the region of individual human development.

These four psychologies fit with what we have come to know about infant and child development as well. Certainly the importance of bodily pleasure experiences and wishes for repetition of those and other satisfactions, the importance of mastery and adaptation, and the importance of relations to significant others are clear observables whose important developmental transformations and elaborations can be traced. Overall, they are what the stuff of development is about. The question of "self" is softer, less readily observable perhaps; but analytically sophisticated infant and child clinical researchers such as René Spitz (1957), Winnicott (1956), and Margaret Mahler (1972) have found the concept indispensable, and it has now become a central organizing concept in more systematic empirical research as well (Stern, 1985). That the terms of the psychologies of drive, ego, object relations, and self have a fit and a utility both in the psychoanalytic situation and in the child-observational one adds to the credence we give them.

A point made by Arnold Cooper (1987a) is relevant here. He wishes to contest an extreme statement of a hermeneutic position in which "there is no other past than the one we construct, and there is no way of understanding the past except through its relation to the present" (p. 83). He goes on to say:

> I would emphasize that psychoanalysis, like history but unlike fiction, does have anchoring points. History's anchoring points are the evidences that events did occur. There was a Roman Empire, it did have dates, actual persons lived and died. These "facts" place a limit on the narratives and interpretations that may seriously be entertained. Psychoanalysis is anchored in its scientific base in developmental psychology and in the biology of attachment and affects. Biology confers limits and regularities on possible histories, and our constructions of the past must accord with this scientific knowledge. Constructions of childhood that are incompatible with what we know of developmental possibilities may open our eyes to new concepts of development, but more likely they alert us to maimed childhoods that have led our patients to unusual narrative constructions in the effort to maintain self-esteem and internal coherence. (pp. 83–84)

The terms of the psychologies of drive, ego, object relations, and self—characterizing the developmental process as they do—are such "anchoring points" for psychoanalysis. And the fact, again, that they characterize individual development "confers limits" on, and offers possibilities for, the "possible histories" that we can construct. (This connects to my comment in the preface that my arguments can be drawn into either side of the current hermeneutics versus science debate. On the one hand, the perspectives from the several standpoints of drive, ego, object, and self can be seen as providing alternative possible narrations or interpretations of the life story; and such indeed they do. But on the other hand, they also provide anchor points in the developmental process that limit and direct the actual narratives that apply, in particular as they apply to this or that individual's specific life history.)

And finally, the fact that the terms of the four psychologies are readily applicable to individual development not only lends them credence for *us* as appropriate abstractions from the flow of clinical material, but also makes them ring true for *patients*. When offered to them via interpretation or reconstruction, patients can readily connect such terms with their life histories as experienced and as expressed in current functioning. As Roy Schafer (1983) points out, we create many narratives, many "tellings" of the life history, with our patients. But I believe these are all likely to be in the terms of one or another of the four psychologies that I have listed, not only because clinical work has taught us of their relevance, but because of their fit with individual history. And not even a more extreme view of the questionable nature of the historical truth that we arrive at in an analysis (such as Spence's, 1982) would argue that *any* random narrative is equally usable; the narrative has to make sense to the patient, and this will be measured against the terms of current and remembered intrapsychic life. In that life, these four psychologies will play central roles.

This leads me to one final point with respect to my decision to work with four psychologies. I shall try for an integrative approach in relation to the four, but one that respects both their differences and their converging contributions. But a different approach could also be taken; that is, the attempt could be made to reduce the four to one or another of them. For three reasons, I reject that approach. First, in the light of the expansion of psychoanalytic theory over the years and the expansion of clinical phenomena seen in the "widening scope" (Stone, 1954) of psychoanalytic work, such attempts at reduction seem to me to be arbitrary; convincing reductionistic views can perhaps be argued, but they can be well argued for more than one of the psychologies. Second, as I shall try to show in chapter 5, the phenomena of each of the four psychologies achieve motivational status over time and function as independent actors on the intrapsychic stage; this enhances their relative independence, at least conceptually. And third, and stemming directly from the points I have been making about individual development, the work of both clinician-observers and empirical researchers on infancy makes clear that the phenomena neither of drive, ego, object relations, nor self experience has a clear primacy in infant life; rather, each has very early origins (and a significant developmental history, I should add—see chapter 4). So at this point it seems to me that the four are not reducible to one another. Taken together they give us both greater range for describing aspects of the clinical situation and greater opportunity to locate a fit between clinical work and developmental history.

A PREVIEW AND A POINT OF VIEW

I shall be working with four sets of phenomena that I subsume under the terms drive, ego, object relations, and self. In the next chapter I discuss each of them in more detail, also discussing a number of issues surrounding the use I make of them. The phenomena are seen both clinically and in the developmental process, and chapters 3 and 4, respectively, focus on each of those two areas. The clinical discussion (chapter 3) is built around the concept "evenly suspended attention" (Freud, 1912), around what we can be attuned to hear in the patient's free associations. And the developmental discussion (chapter 4) is built around the argument that both early core developments and continuing lifelong ones occur with respect to each of the four psychologies. Finally, chapters 5 and 6 treat of some larger theoretical questions: the question of motivation in each of the psychologies and of the organization of the personality across all four of them, respectively.

Part II of the book is devoted entirely to examples of the phenomena of the four psychologies as drawn from the clinical situation. In chapter 7 this is approached through process notes of individual sessions, and in chapter 8 through summaries of completed analyses. The clinical examples are meant to be mundane in a certain sense—that is, they should seem unsurprising and familiar. My argument is that phenomena of each of the psychologies inevitably surface in any analysis and are addressed interpretively. My aim is to tease them apart conceptually to highlight the range of work that goes into any analysis—notwithstanding that not all of it may get represented in the theories any particular analyst uses. The four psychologies are conceptually separable, and to a degree separable in our descriptions of development, though dynamically and structurally thoroughly integrated in any clinical instance.

And finally, in part III, I shall present a series of applications of the ideas presented herein: a diagnostic/developmental exploration of the concept "preoedipal pathology" and the related concept "ego defect" (chapters 9 and 10); a discussion of the current debates over the concept of a symbiotic phase, and of the phase concept in general (chapter 11); and a clinical exploration of the mutative factors in psychoanalysis and dynamic psychotherapy (chapter 12). All of these can have light shed on them when viewed from a four psychologies standpoint.

When I have discussed and presented these ideas earlier, the questions came up: is it legitimate to think of these as four psychologies of *psychoanalysis?* is this not such a hodgepodge that it no longer deserves that name? I do not think so. I believe that each of the four, and especially the four taken together, require just such a complex and multifaceted view of human functioning as only psychoanalysis provides.

Freud (1914a) defined psychoanalysis, in the clinical situation, as a treatment that centers on the analysis of resistance and transference; and nothing about the varied phenomena of the four psychologies requires any change in that view. Freud, however, never did define psychoanalytic theory in any such singleminded way. Quite the reverse, at least insofar as his drive psychology was concerned. He explicitly recognized that "the witch, metapsychology" (1937) and his formulations regarding instinct theory were the dispensable mythology of psychoanalytic theory (1915). Such concepts could come and go; only *observation* provided the bedrock—and the evolution of just that clinical observation has produced the four psychologies.

And I believe that the four are consistent with the core of psychoanalysis, even in its traditional form. Thus, separately and jointly, the four psychologies share the assumptions of *psychic determinism,* of *unconscious mental functioning,* and of (for want of a better term) the *primary process*—that aspect of thinking that is based on symbol and metaphor, on "irrational" connections among ideas, and that does not heed the rules of reality and social communication. Only by following the premises underlying this triad of psychic phenomena can we find our way to the place of the phenomena of each of the four psychologies in the lives of our patients. Furthermore, the four psychologies all work with core psychoanalytic assumptions, which state that individual character is shaped by early, bodily based, and object-related experiences, all organized in interconnected (both multiply functional and conflictual) ways. The bodily based experiences of drive and gratification, of apparatus and function, are among the contents thus organized, as are the object-tied experiences involved in drive gratification, the learning of modes of psychological (ego) functioning, the creation and growth of the self experience, and the shaping of the world of object representations (Sandler and Rosenblatt, 1962). So I think they are indeed four psychologies of psychoanalysis, and as such they find places in each psychoanalytic treatment within the traditional boundaries of quiet listening, work with resistance and transference, and the clinical triad of neutrality, abstinence, and relative anonymity.

But I do not wish to argue that they simply fit into or are coterminous with the traditional confines of psychoanalysis. Rather, as I shall develop them, they require us to see psychoanalysis not only as a psychology of conflict but also of repetition and of development, the last with all of the attendant delays and aberrations that are inherent in any developmental process; all three are omnipresent in the clinical situation. The use of the four psychologies in clinical work, I believe, provides a fuller approximation to the phenomena of clinical psychoanalysis (including reconstructed individual histories) than any one or two alone. And they are responsive to the clinical material that cultural changes and changing psychopathology in contemporary patients have brought our way.

Nothing in what I have just pointed to as the traditional core of psychoanalytic theory has to do with specific substantive contents of the mind or of development. These contents, I contend, can and do vary widely, and the array of contents addressed by the several psychologies captures those that we have, in our clinical work, thus far found to be significant. But in addressing such a wide range of contents, I come to the second criticism that I have had leveled against these ideas as I began to develop them—namely, that they represent nothing but eclecticism; "mere" eclecticism is usually implied.

Aside from the fact that eclecticism need not be "mere," eclecticism is not in fact my intent. Recall that I shall in no way be attempting to draw together different theories (such as Fairbairn's, 1941; Kohut's, 1977; Hartmann's, 1939). Rather, I shall be attempting to evolve a structure that can give representation to the diverse array of phenomena that analysts in fact work with, and to spell out a unifying view. Having attempted (in chapters 1–5) to make a convincing case for the significance of phenomena from the domains of the four psychologies, I shall (in chapter 6) present a relatively simple set of organizing ideas for encompassing them all. In a sense, that organizing structure can be seen as a "content-free" theory. It deals with units of development and the ways in which they become interrelated and integrated in the construction of that complex formation that we call the individual personality. But in principle any contents could provide the initial units that become the building blocks of personality; in that sense, the view is content-free. But, of course, and in fact, the biological, early nurturing, and general cultural commonalities among all humankind make certain contents central for each of us; they are not accidental. But they are diverse. And this is the ultimate reason for my working with this wide array of phenomena; the manysidedness of people as we come to know them clinically requires it, and many of the extant theories tilt in one direction or another more heavily than the evidence supports.

If one were stranded on a desert isle, it would probably be better to find there a set of tools than, say, a finished house. The house would indeed provide shelter from the start, but the tools could be used flexibly in innumerable ways—including the building of a house—to enhance the capacity to get along. I view what I have been calling the four psychologies of psychoanalysis as just such tools to be used flexibly when one is stranded in the position of analytic listener. They do not provide, at the start, a finished house—a full theoretical structure—but they are, I find, immensely useful to help one get along in doing analysis. It is in this sense that the phenomena I shall describe and their varying assemblages that I shall propose should be understood.

The classical Freudian theory has been built around specific contents and concepts (though, as noted, I do not see these as its core)—notably the instinctual drives and the organization of the mind along the lines of the tripartite structural model. But there is additionally a classical Freudian *intent*—that is, the search for in-depth understanding of human mental life. I hope I am true to that intent. For me, the relevant question is not, is this psychoanalysis? but, is it useful clinically? and can it be incorporated into the general psychoanalytic way of thinking? Those questions are arguable; but they are the relevant questions. I believe that a view of the person in terms of a wide array of significant centers and forms of psychological activity, developing an equally wide array of central motives, and organized in complex individualized ways (personal hierarchies of the four psychologies, I shall call them) not only reflects human function with some accuracy but in fact underlies the actual day-to-day work of clinical psychoanalysis.

CHAPTER 2

The Four Psychologies of Psychoanalysis

IN HIS PAPER "Metapsychology as a Multimodel System," Pinchas Noy (1977) writes:

> My basic hypothesis . . . is that the uniqueness of psychoanalysis is in its metapsychology which is based on a multimodel theoretical system, i.e., a system composed of several theoretical models. In this respect it differs from almost all other contemporary schools in psychology and behavioral sciences, each one of which is based on a single and uniform model. The existence of these numerous models enables us to arrange clinical raw data in several alternate patterns, allowing the examination of each phenomenon from several points of view and the transfer of the focus of interest from one point of view to another, according to the specific clinical, experimental, or theoretical needs. The fact that there exists no single unifying basic theoretical model from which all psycho-analytic facts, hypotheses, and interventions are to be derived, is not a

weakness, as is commonly regarded in science, but it is the outstanding feature of psychoanalysis and the source of its specific power to survive and adapt. (p. 1)

He goes on to compare this to the familiar example of light understood as both waves and particles and, drawing on David Rapaport and Merton Gill's (1959) paper on the five metapsychological points of view, he suggests that we now have "seven models which are more or less accepted: the dynamic, economic, topographic, psychogenetic, structural, adaptive, and psychosocial models" (1977, p. 4). In the remainder of his paper, Noy goes on to say that models are merely tools for thinking, that we should be cautious to avoid reifying them, and that new data will stretch the models beyond their point of usefulness and will ultimately require the development of new models.

It is in the general spirit of all of Noy's remarks that I work with the four psychologies here. Taking them together, I believe, we have another route to the "specific power [of psychoanalysis] to survive and adapt." I do note, however, that at least the first six of the seven models he lists (I am not sure what he refers to, specifically, with the "psychosocial" model) were developed in relation to what I would call the drive psychology. Clearly, I slice the models pie another way.

I believe that people have urges, have relations to others that derive from (often distorted) memories that they carry within, have modes of what we call defense and adaptation, and have subjective experiences that we consensually think of as "my *self*." But in spite of the reality of such phenomena, there is no question that it is virtually impossible to say anything about them without having constructed a model. What passes for description—indeed, the very choice of things to describe—involves prior theoretical choices and preconceptions (Schafer, 1986). Though I aim in general for experience-near descriptions of phenomena, it is clear that the whole enterprise is governed by larger and smaller models of human behavior. So I carve the behavioral pie into four psychologies, with recognition that there are overlaps among them and that, within each, a case can often be made for further subdivision. Ultimately, my interest in these psychologies, specifically as a differentiable yet interconnected foursome, has come about through the help they offer in clinical work; they expand pathways both to the understanding of clinical data and to the evolution of clinical technique. My interest in them arose pragmatically, through asking, what furthers the analytic work and produces patient change?

I do not mean to suggest that psychoanalysis has heretofore ignored any of these several points of view. While the drive and ego perspectives on individual functioning were more formally part of Freud's theory, psychoanalytic practice clearly deals with them all. Early object relations and their repetition are significant parts of the working stuff of any analysis, and the ongoing subjective state is always a touchstone for the in-session work. All four are by now well established in aspects of the psychoanalytic literature. I describe them as four psychologies because I believe each generates different questions about our clinical work (chapter 3), because distinctive motivational features develop in each (chapter 5), and because each can play a varyingly central role in the overall organization of the personality (chapter 6). It is useful to grant each of the psychologies a place in our minds, as I hope to show.

DEVELOPMENTS IN THE
PSYCHOANALYTIC LITERATURE

From a current perspective, the growth of both the clinical and developmental theories of psychoanalysis can be seen as having taken place in three waves—drive psychology, ego psychology, and object relations theory—with the last producing an interest in the self (in contradistinction to the object) as well. To a considerable degree, the evolution of these ideas is based on new modes or domains of observation: the use of free association and the couch, the turn to child analysis and then to infant and child observation, and the "widening scope" of patients worked with in analysis later on (Stone, 1954). These developments, plus new observations within the standard clinical psychoanalytic situation, led to new formulations. But additionally, the roles of individual contributors, perhaps specifically attuned to one or another aspect of human function because of their personal life histories, cannot be ignored.

The first wave, drive psychology, was initiated by Freud's abandonment of the seduction theory (1897) and his articulation of the theory of infantile sexuality (1905) and led to the early mushrooming of writings on drives,

their manifold transformations, and their role in psychopathology. It is certainly no accident that the first great formulations of psychoanalysis were
those having to do with instinctual drives. Freud came of age scientifically in
a time of Newtonian, physicalistic science (Holt, 1972), a world of force and
counterforce, within which his ideas regarding instinct and repressive barriers, cathexes and countercathexes, readily fit. Further, Freud was born into
the world of middle-class Middle Europe in the repressive, antisexual culture of the mid- and late nineteenth century. The personal organizing issues
for him (as discovered in his self-analysis) and for his patients, those that
took center stage when the free-associative process was first undertaken,
were those of sexuality (especially) and, more broadly, of urge, of social and
internalized taboo, and hence of conflict, defense, anxiety, guilt, defensive
failure, and symptom formation. But additionally, Freud was born into a
more or less intact family with reasonably reliable (even if conflicted) relationships; hence the kinds of inner formations and life experiences that we
might today conceptualize in terms of defect in ego function or early failures of object contact and core identification were not centrally part of his
personal experience and psychopathology. Furthermore, his progressive
clarification of patient suitability for both the rigors and potentials of psychoanalytic treatment led him to exclude those with defective ego function (for
example, those whose intrapsychic defenses and observer capacity could not
be called upon reliably to work with the anxieties triggered by the psychoanalytic process or those for whom free association tended to lead to excessive
loosening of thought organization) or those with faulted early object experience (for example, where a transference neurosis could not develop or
where the patient could not stand the isolation and abstinence of the analytic posture and conduct on the couch). These exclusions restricted his access to these forms of pathology and the demands they would make upon
developmental and clinical theory.

In the history of the development of ideas, these limitations of focus have
to be viewed as fortunate for the development of psychoanalysis as theory.
No science and no scientist can study the whole problem in any area at
once. Only by narrowing focus (and ordinarily, as well, by having conceptual organizers for the narrowed area under study) does a science progress.
And Freud's early discoveries in drive psychology proved stimulating
enough to further the growth of psychoanalysis as theory and treatment
method for its first three to four decades. The formulations regarding in-

stincts and their vicissitudes (1915); the earliest formulations regarding character largely in terms of the widening and defended-against life of the drives (Freud, 1908; Abraham, 1921, 1924); a view of defense early on in terms of the vicissitudes of drive (1915) and ultimately in terms of conflict with drive; the understanding of what is resisted by the resistance, of what is repeated in the transference, and of those fixated and pent-up forces that power the analytic work itself; a developmental theory formulated around psychosexual stages and the forms of the tie to the object that are consequent upon movement through those stages—all these testify to the seminal nature of Freud's earliest drive-based psychology. The potential in this area of theory formation was enough to absorb the creative energy of the first generation of analysts for years.

But clinical observations and the requirements of theoretical clarity did not allow things to rest at this point. In retrospect it can be seen that even the early drive psychology was not articulated without a conception of what later came to be called the ego and of its specific functions. Certainly Freud needed a conception of defense (repression) from the outset. And his theory of dreams (1900) could not help but deal with the nature of the *thought* process and its role as a detour route to satisfaction, the rise to *perceptual* intensity of the dream, the *inhibition of motility* during sleep—all aspects of human function that later achieved a central role in psychoanalytic theory under the term *ego apparatuses*, inborn and a potential base for ego development (Freud, 1937; Hartmann, 1939), the guarantors of autonomy from the drives (Rapaport, 1957), and having pervasive developmental and functional ties to those drives.

These were some of the early seeds of an ego psychology. Later developments pushed the theory along in that same direction. Many clinical observations contributed: (1) adaptation was an observable fact of life, and the capacity of individuals to deal with adversity and to make something creative and constructive out of conflict could not go unnoticed by the analysts who were working close up with these individuals; (2) psychoanalytic treatment could rest with analysis (Freud, 1919) because the work of synthesis and integration, notwithstanding the place of working through (Freud, 1914b), seemed to be a native feature of human function; (3) character, forged out of drives and their transformation (Freud, 1908; Abraham, 1921, 1924), turned out to be a major adaptive (vis-à-vis the outside) and regulating (vis-à-vis the inside) achievement in personal organization and development and not only a vicissitude of drive; and (4) the observation that anxiety seemed to precede (and hence signal) defense rather than to follow repression (as a transformation of libido into anxiety) (Freud, 1926) led to a conception of a much more powerful ego that could, via the anxiety signal, call the pleasure-pain principle into play against the drives in a situation of conflict.

The work of the early child analysts and child observers, especially Anna Freud (1926, 1936), also contributed to the press toward an ego psychology, because childhood is, par excellence, a time of the rapid development of new modes of mastery, of (under fortunate circumstances) creative resolutions of conflict, of the development of skills and interests that themselves foster adaptation, conflict resolution, and self-esteem. No child observer or therapist can fail to be impressed with the side of the person that manages, copes, or even simply muddles through: the ego. And drive theory, the unconscious, and later (Freud, 1923) the theory of the id itself created a need for an ego theory. For if the id does not learn, if the unconscious is timeless, how can human adaptation and mastery be derived solely from them? Some conception of an inborn learning-and-adaptation structure (that is, the ego apparatuses) or a process by which drive energies could be transformed in their function (that is, neutralized [Hartmann, 1955; Kris, 1955]) was needed to account for the clear observables of human development off the couch—in life.

And so Freud developed a formal theory of the ego as one of the tripartite systems of the mind (1923), expanded it (1926) in a reformulation that led to a "strong" ego concept (not merely one that rode the "horse"— reality, drive, conscience—in the direction it wanted to go but one that could steer it), and was followed in this area by others who made major systematic contributions (A. Freud, 1936; Hartmann, 1939). The result is a theory of the ego, its development, and its functions; a conception of autonomy, adaptation, and the conflict-free sphere; as well as a conception (even if not fully articulated) of the characteristics of ego function requisite in a patient who undertakes an analysis. And so the second wave, ego psychology, reached its crest.

In a certain sense, the conceptual work of these first two waves represents an attempt to recognize the biology of the organism in psychological theory. The individual is seen as starting with various biological givens. Taking those that have central relevance for the developing psychology of the person, we divide them conceptually into the drives (represented in urges, leading to wishes and fantasies) and the ego (the apparatuses, from which grow capabilities for defense, adaptation, and reality testing). But there also exist those things, significant for the psychological development of the individual, that stem from relationships with others. In fact, the contrasting views of a person's development that are addressed in psychoanalytic drive theory, on the one hand, or object relations theory, on the other, represent the psychoanalytic rendition of the familiar nature-nurture controversy. Implicitly they ask, how much (and in what ways) can individual development be seen as determined by inborn, biologically based drives (and the equally inborn modifiers that we call ego apparatuses) and how much by experienced relations with others? This third wave, the study of object relations, is still very much propelling us and so is more difficult to see in perspective. It is clear, however, that in the way our theories have evolved attention to a self has gone hand in hand with attention to the object. Let us turn to this whole region now.

In spite of the centrality of drive concepts in classical psychoanalytic theories of human development and pathogenesis, a major part of any clinical psychoanalysis has to do with the patient's contemporary and remembered relations with significant others. A lot of free-association time is devoted to such relationships. We teach patients, so to speak, through interpretation, the power of lasting urges in their lives—urges that underlie inhibitions, symptoms, and anxiety; urges that produce endlessly repetitive maladaptive behavior; urges that are expressed in dreams and fantasies, in character traits, in interests and vocations. And we show them how, through the action of their lasting urges and specific wishes, they themselves shape the very relationships that distress and plague them. But nonetheless patients teach us the significance of others. We get some sense of the alternative possibilities *in reality* offered by different relationships, even though we can never be certain of the veridicality of what we hear. And we certainly hear of patients' preoccupation with relationships.

Theoretical developments followed clinical observations. The formal movement toward an intrapsychic (rather than interpersonal) object relations theory, and for its essential unity with drive psychology—both conditions ensuring its tie to the mainstream of psychoanalysis—was implicit in the writings of Melanie Klein and of Fairbairn. Klein (1921–1945) spoke of early *drive* processes (libidinal and destructive) in terms of the incorporation and expulsion of good and bad *objects*, thus cementing the tie (or actually creating a certain equivalence) of drive and object. And Fairbairn (1941), coining the term *object relations theory* and emphasizing the object-seeking (rather than pleasure-seeking) nature of the libidinal drives, also cemented the conceptual tie of drive and object. Though Freud (1915), too, had spoken of the object in terms that tied it to drive—the object being that thing through which satisfaction is achieved—Fairbairn's shift in emphasis and in the concept of the object was significant. The focus moves away from object as secondary to satisfaction and toward the primacy of object seeking in itself. The concept of the object changes along with this, for it is not simply nipple, or thumb, or teddy bear (that is, anything that serves to satisfy drive) that is conceived of as object but rather the whole significant primary caretaker at the outset and later others.

But it remained for a new mode of observation to become significant—in this case direct infant and child observation—for object relations theory to achieve its greatest impetus. Thus, Winnicott's whole body of work (1958b, 1965) provides a bridge between Klein's and Fairbairn's work and later contributions. Based as it is on close-up observation of mothers and infants and on his unique attempt to imagine his way into their experience, and formulated largely in object-relational terms (bridging the interpersonal and the intrapsychic), Winnicott's work can be seen as an attempt to bring Klein's reconstructive concepts down to earth, anchoring them in possible (even though still only imagined or inferred) actual mother-infant experiences. From this point of view, Klein's error lay not in turning to inferred or imagined phenomena of the earliest months but in dragging oedipal and superego concepts along as she did so rather than abandoning them for that period. Winnicott did what Klein failed to do, speaking of destructive and incorporative processes in terms closer to the observables and inferables of the mother-infant dyad.

Once the turn to child observation took place, the focus on object relations was inevitable. The psychoanalytic situation, especially with the neurotic patient, is one that readily supports the view that the patient's life is largely of his or her own making. Barring the prototypic situation of a safe falling off a roof onto a person's head, a patient's "fate," including "accidents," and certainly ongoing inner experiences and object relations, seems to entail endless experiences of, or repetitions of, what he or she brings along intrapsychically. A focus on wish, fantasy, and character rather than on what others do to the patient leads to the most effective psychoanalytic work. What we see is the powerful impact of wish and fantasy; we only hear about the role of other persons. But in child (especially infant) observations exactly the reverse obtains. The powerful shaping influence of the primary caretaker, the opportunities, deprivations, satisfactions, and models she (and others) provide, is what even the psychoanalytic observer sees most readily; in contrast, the very young child's inner life is essentially unavailable to us, except via inference. The growing child-observational tradition among analysts thus gives support to theoretical formulations regarding the primacy of the object in development. Analysts who, as clinicians, were organizing the data of lives around urges and wishes were, as infant researchers, now organizing those data around infant-caretaker interactions, resulting ultimately in an expansion of theory. John Bowlby's (1969, 1973, 1980) work as well, influenced also by ethological research, falls into this broad tradition and has culminated in his emphasis on the object-related concepts of attachment and separation.

Two areas of clinical work, at varying distances from the mainstream of psychoanalysis, also led to formulations emphasizing the role of the other in the development of the individual. In each, new clinical observations, stemming essentially from the difficulty in understanding the development of psychopathology primarily from a drive-defense standpoint, led to these object-related formulations. First, clinicians who had substantial contact with schizophrenics (Sullivan, 1953; Fromm-Reichmann, 1950) developed interpersonal theories that, while by no means equivalent to what has come to be called object relations theory within psychoanalysis, nonetheless pointed the way to the significance of the *other*. That the interpersonal view arose at least in part out of work with schizophrenics reflects the by now widely held view that the earliest object relationships were somehow faulty for these individuals. Freud's consideration of the "narcissistic neuroses" in which transference would not be formed reflects his observation that something is basically wrong in the connectedness of such patients to others. As the data base (here schizophrenia versus neurosis) varies, so too do the explanatory formulations (exactly as child observation and psychoanalytic treatment produce different data and therefore somewhat varying formulations). The second clinical development, more recent and arguably closer to the mainstream, is in Heinz Kohut's (1971, 1977) work, where, again, encounters with a clinical population somewhat different from the classical neurotic patient led to formulations centering on a "self" and to a developmental theory heavily weighting the confirming/mirroring/rewarding inputs of the *other*.

For Freud (1915), the position of the object was defined as the end point in the search for gratification. The very term *object* (rather than *person*) clearly reflects that the "thing" through which gratification is achieved could be a person but could also be a part of a person (thumb, breast) or an inanimate object (blanket, bottle, or, as in fetishism, say, an item of clothing). By and large, this is not the case for object relations theory. The object is a person or his or her representation, with varying degrees of veridicality based upon distortion by drive and defensive processes. So object relations theory has come to refer to internal mental representations of self and other (Sandler and Rosenblatt, 1962) in varying experienced and ideal forms, bound together by affects (Kernberg, 1976), memories, and behavioral expectancies, and having a determinative influence upon current functioning. What defines contemporary object relations theory is not simply the primacy of object relatedness, as proposed initially by Fairbairn (1941)—for drive satisfaction and object relation rapidly become interwoven—but a view of mental life that is organized around self and object representations and their relations and repetitions in addition to an organization of mental life around drive, defense, and conflict.

Historically, in the psychoanalytic literature, attention to the self has been an offshoot of attention to relationships between self and other. First Spitz (1957) focused on the cognitive differentiation of the "me" from the "not me," the self from the other. In a long series of works, Mahler (see 1966; Mahler et al., 1975) added to the understanding of this cognitive differentiation and especially of its affective consequences. Winnicott, steeped in observations of infants with mothers, also came to develop ideas regarding an emerging self—for example, the "going on being" (Winnicott, 1956) of the infant, which produces the core of a self, and the beginning of authenticity (the "true" self) when the infant's spontaneous gestures are adequately met by the environment so that inner impulse gets to be expressible in relation to the outer world (Winnicott, 1960a). And, more recently, Kohut (1971, 1977) has developed his focus on the self in a view in which it is entrenched in the role of the other as (for example, mirroring and/or idealized) selfobject. All of these theorists inextricably link theoretical attention to the self with attention to relationships with others. Altogether they have produced an array of concepts having to do with the differentiation, affective tone, integrity, and authenticity of the self.

Thus, developments in the literature have produced concepts that address phenomena of drive, ego, object relations, and self. This has not taken place, however, without major competitive conceptual battles, sometimes with the lines between ad hominem argument and theoretical argument becoming blurred. The emergence of an ego psychology has been seen at times and by some as a move toward "acceptability" and away from the powerful but threatening formulations regarding sexual and aggressive drives. And object relations theories, too, have been variously seen as putting the cart before the horse (object relations before drive) or, by their sometimes emphasis on the earliest object relations, as distorting (by placing too early) or discounting (by focusing on early events) the centrality of the oedipus complex. Drive theory, in its turn, has been seen as representing a conceptual attachment to outdated mechanistic/energic notions. And most recently, Kohut's (1977) particular psychology of the self has been attacked for negating drive and conflict and being too environmental in its emphasis (a criticism also leveled against object relations theory at times), while in turn it has viewed the drive psychology as subordinate to the "superordinate" theory of the self within which drive conflicts are merely "disintegration products," that is, symptoms of primary disorders of the self.

These theoretical differences are generally reflected in contrasting views—preferences and insights—of one or another theorist regarding clinical psychopathology and the forms of its making (and unmaking, through treatment) and in the sometimes explicit and sometimes silent assumptions about development and pathogenesis that are carried into the clinical situation. Yet there seems to me to be no doubt that many a theorist and many a working clinician experiences these expansions in theory as together producing rich new possibilities for encompassing the vicissitudes of the developmental process and the exigencies of clinical work.

FOUR PSYCHOANALYTIC PSYCHOLOGIES

Each of the psychologies views human functioning from a somewhat different perspective and therefore highlights somewhat different aspects of that functioning.

Drive

From the standpoint of the psychology of drive, the individual is seen in terms of the vicissitudes of, and struggles with, lasting urges. These are initially forged in the crucible of early bodily and family experience, but of course undergo modifications as the person moves developmentally through oedipal, childhood, adolescent, and adult phases. From the perspective of the drive psychology, then, the person is and carries the history of his or her encounter with such inner urges. These urges are seen as (1) ultimately biologically based but achieving psychological representation and form; (2) unfolding according to a preprogrammed epigenetic sequence, yet susceptible to profound disruptions and alterations of this program in the complex organism that the human being is; and (3) subject to near endless varieties of transformation via delay, displacement, sublimation, and other defensive and expressive vicissitudes, such that their currently active forms and their presumed origins do not stand in any clear one-to-one relationship to each other. That the basic drives Freud worked with in his final dual instinct theory were sexuality and aggression is, of course, well known, but is also in a certain sense secondary to the core position of the drive psychology— namely, that *some* lasting urges, undergoing modification and transformation, have lifelong effects and must be understood adequately to understand current behavior.

In any event, such biologically based urges ultimately take the form of psychological wishes that may or may not be embodied in actions but are certainly embodied in conscious or unconscious fantasies. Because many of these wishes come to be experienced as unacceptable and dangerous, psychic life is seen as organized around conflict and its resolution— signified by anxiety, guilt, aspects of shame, inhibition, symptom formation, and pathological character traits. In this picture, guilt has a special place. For conscience, from the perspective of the drive psychology, is seen in part as a vicissitude of aggressive drive, turned on the self, based on identifications with the nay-saying parents, and fostering control of urge through the cognition/affect of guilt. Though psychoanalysis has produced a metapsychological theory of instinctual drive, at the experiential level of human functioning that I shall be addressing here the focus is on wish and urge, defense against them, and conflict (see Holt, 1976; G. S. Klein, 1976).

Ego

Historically, as already described, a psychology of ego function took its major thrust from the drive-conflict psychology and remains intimately tied to it via the conception of (ego) defense against drive. But later, Hartmann's (1939) work introduced a significant emphasis on adaptation to the average expectable environment as well. I propose now that, overall, from the standpoint of the psychology of the ego, the individual is seen in terms of capacities for adaptation, reality testing, and defense and their use in the clinical situation and in life at large to deal with the inner world of urges, affects, and fantasies and the outer world of reality demands. So the whole sphere of learning, as well as defense, is encompassed here, though our interest in learning, as analysts, is likely to be most centrally from the perspective of its role in the modification and the handling by the individual of his or her significant intrapsychic issues.

Developmentally, the capacities for adaptation, reality testing, and defense are seen as slowly attained and expanding over time: they are a result of learning. Such a developmental conception of ego functioning allows also for significant emphasis on a concept of ego defect. That is, since adults (and older children) have capacities for adaptation, reality testing, and defense that infants do not have, we have to assume that these developed in between. Anything that develops can develop poorly or in aberrant ways, and those developmental failures that occur in the domain of adaptive capacities can be viewed as ego defects. I have in mind, as examples, such things as affect intolerance and flooding, unreliable delay and control over impulses, and failure to obtain object constancy. Such defects are not unrelated to conflict; conflict may have been contributory to their going wrong developmentally, and they will in any case enter into the individual's fantasy life and self experience and hence become elements in conflict and take on multiple functions (Waelder, 1936). But I believe they can also usefully (from a working clinical standpoint) be seen as defects—adaptational incapacities or faulted capacities (see chapter 10).

Object Relations

From the standpoint of the psychology of object relations, the individual is seen in terms of an internal drama, derived from early childhood, that is carried around within as memory (conscious or unconscious) and in which the individual enacts one or more or all of the roles (see Sandler and Rosenblatt, 1962). These internal images, loosely based on childhood experiences, also put their stamp on new experience, so that these in turn are assimilated to the old dramas rather than being experienced fully in their contemporary form. These internal dramas are understood to be formed out of experiences with the primary objects of childhood, but are not seen as veridical representations of those relationships. The object relation *as experienced* by the child is what is laid down in memory and repeated, and this experience is a function of the affect and wishes active in the child at the moment of the experience. Thus, illustratively and hypothetically, the same quietly pensive and inactive mother will be experienced as a depriver by the hungry child, but perhaps as comfortingly in tune by the child who is contentedly playing alone. Significant for the clinical relevance of the object relations psychology is the tendency to repeat these old family dramas, a repetition propelled by efforts after attachment or after mastery or both. From the perspective of this view of the object relations psychology, one aspect of pathology is seen in the degree to which perceptions of current reality, and the actualities of current behavior, are determined by internally carried representations from the past rather than by current actuality. The more this is so, the more pathology; the less, the less. A second perspective on pathology stemming from this viewpoint is, obviously, in the nature of the particular internal dramas carried around and lived out.

Freud, too, had his object relations theory, though he did not conceptualize it in those terms. The formal status he gave to the object was drive based—that is, the object was that person, part of a person, part of the self, or thing through which gratification of drive was attained. But in at least three of his major contributions he went far toward what later came to be central to object relations concepts. I am referring, first, to his views regarding *identification*—specifically to his formulation that all significant object relations, when lost, are replaced by an identification, thus leaving a mark upon the ego (Freud, 1917). Through identification we retain an inner, lived-out, relation to the significant persons of our past. This can be seen as the product of oral incorporative tendencies linked to need (that is, to drives) and/or to inborn originally autonomous, tools of learning that fulfill their evolutionary function in enabling such within-species learning to take place. But in either event, the concept of identification, and the pervasiveness of the phenomena to which it refers, opens the door wide to the significance of the object in the course of human development. Second, the *oedipus complex* itself, for Freud the pivotal fulcrum of development—the place where preoedipal phenomena achieve a new organization and where the person's course is set into the future—is itself equally susceptible to description as a stage in the development of the child's sexual (and, here, possessive, rivalrous, and aggressive) wishes or as a powerful and formative set of triangular object relations that has its roots in the human family structure. It is not one or the other; it is both. And in either case, it eventuates in further identifications, here especially the one that we refer to as the formation of conscience—the superego. And the third of Freud's concepts that I shall mention here with regard to its object relational implications is *transference*. This living out of personal history in the relation to, and on the person of, the analyst—so central to clinical work—is, again, equally susceptible to description as the result of the continuous press of drives toward discharge or as the result of a universal tendency toward repetition of old object relationships, based not only on their pleasure, but on their traumatic nature "beyond the pleasure principle," in efforts at control and mastery. That these and other concepts of Freud's can be viewed in drive and/or object relational terms simply reflects the fact of overdetermination and multiple function in human life—that is, it speaks to human complexity.

Self

Let me now turn, last and with most trepidation, to a psychology of self experience. I am not here referring to Kohut's (1977) formal Self Psychology. Kohut's is a view that has at least three major components: it is a psychology of subjective states of the person; it is a developmental psychology built largely around parental inputs; and it is a psychology that dictates particular technical interventions in treatment that have a certain supportive-experiential quality much of the time. While I do not intend to cast out what he and others writing in this domain have offered, it is nonetheless only the first of these points—a psychology of subjective states of the person—to which I shall be referring. I seek to emphasize this by referring to a psychology of *self experience* (rather than *the* self); I intend this usage additionally to bypass some problems of conceptualization and to avoid dangers of reification of the self. Subjective self experiences, as I see them, are of course analyzable—in the sense of being reducible to earlier experience, to conflict, to fantasy—and can be productively seen as compromise formations. Nonetheless, I believe these subjective states take on a psychological force, a motivational power, of their own (see chapter 5) and thus take on a causal role. They then have to be addressed clinically at their own level of developmentally attained organization, whether reducible or not. Sheldon Bach (1987) nicely captures an aspect of the issue:

> The ego is a scientific fantasy of the psychoanalyst. . . . It provides an impartial, objective, structurally equidistant and dispassionate view of the person or object of our scrutiny and investigation, a view, as it were, from the moon. The self [by contrast], in its common usage, is an experiential construct. It integrates observations made upon the subject's experience from a phenomenological point of view. . . . The self provides a partisan, subjective, and impassioned view of the person as the perceiver of his own experience. The self is one pole of a phenomenological rather than an intrapsychic theory, the other pole being the object.

The psychology of self experience, as I shall work with it, is a polyglot. It draws on phenomena called to our attention by clinician-theorists of many different outlooks, who point up many and varied phenomena. But what binds them together is their relation to the ongoing subjective state which itself comes to have motive power in individual function. It could well be argued that there are in fact several disparate psychologies of self experience, each of the aspects of my polyglot in fact being a separable psychology. I would not want to argue too forcefully against that view. Indeed, a similar argument about multiplicity of the psychologies could be made with regard to drive, ego, and object relations as well. Certainly sexual and aggressive drives are not seen as following parallel developmental courses; a psychology of ego defect may well deserve to be separated from a psychology of ego defense; and there are numerous differentiable object relations views in the literature (including those of Klein, 1921–1945; Fairbairn, 1941; Kernberg, 1976) which I will not be addressing in any major way. Certainly I recognize a certain arbitrariness in my particular groupings of the four psychologies.

With these considerations as background, then, from the standpoint of the psychology of self experience the individual is seen in terms of the ongoing subjective state, particularly with regard to issues of boundaries, authenticity, agency, and affective tone. In listing these, I am drawing from the current literature those features that have been most impressive to me in my clinical work. Thus, degree of differentiation of self from other has a central place, and here I refer to the sense of separateness, of boundaries (Mahler et al., 1975; Pine, 1979b) or contrariwise, of loss or absence of boundaries. By *authenticity* I refer to the phenomena that Winnicott (1960a) sought to capture in his distinction between true and false self. By *agency* I refer to a person's sense of ability to live his or her own life as an active agent, not "lived" by inner forces or remembrances (see G. S. Klein, 1976; Schafer, 1983) or even the right to have a life (Modell, 1984). And, by the affective tone of the self experience, I refer to Kohut's work (1977) on the degree of wholeness or fragmentation, continuity or discontinuity, or esteem of the self. To varying degrees, most of these areas have to do with the relation of self to other, whether via differentiation from the "dual-unity" (Mahler, 1972), or the parental response to the child's "spontaneous gesture" that allows genuineness to be maintained (Winnicott, 1960a) or the contemporary selfobject serving functions for the self (Kohut, 1977), or the actual historical (mirroring and ideal-forming) functions served by the parent for the child. These all have the ring of connection to those early stages in the development of the self that Daniel Stern (1985) refers to as "self with other." And they remind us of Spitz's (1957) earlier description of the development of the "I" inherently in relation to the "non-I" and, later, of the self in relation to the object. To a large degree the domain of the psychology of self experience is subjective experience specifically with respect to self-definition in relation to the object.

The four psychologies as described are clearly overlapping. Thus, when Self Psychologists describe excited grandiosity or the need for mirroring essentially as efforts toward self-regulation, they are thinking in terms of functions still incompletely or unsuccessfully performed by the self and reflecting sometimes problematic historical or contemporary use of the selfobject; clearly these problems of self-regulation are addressed in the ego psychology as well, through ideas regarding the development of intrapsychic defense. And the role of the object appears prominently in the self and object relations psychologies as I use them. In the former, however, its role has to do with incomplete, aberrant, or otherwise problematic differentiation from the object, whereas in the latter it has to do with internalized object relations (Kernberg, 1976)—that is, with an internal drama derived from childhood that is carried around within and in which the individual enacts one or more or all of the roles (Sandler and Rosenblatt, 1962); the drive psychology, too, of course, works with the object concept—as the end point in the search for gratification. From another standpoint, the idea of wished for role relationships (Sandler and Sandler, 1978) ties together the drive and object relations psychologies in a particularly compelling way. And, yet again, the superego concept must be addressed at least through the concepts of a drive psychology (the oedipus complex and the special role of aggression) and an object relations psychology (internalization, identification). These overlaps notwithstanding, I believe it is useful to distinguish among the several psychologies conceptually, as I shall try to demonstrate in subsequent chapters.

Priorities among the four psychologies can be argued. Does the nature of early object relations lead to particular functional drive constellations? or do variations in fundamental drive strength color the object relations to begin with? Are self experiences laid down, or are ego functions formed, in quiescent moments, independent of drive? or as by-products of drive-dominated moments? or both? While such issues can be debated, I shall instead work from two other positions. First that, however initiated, phenomena of drive, ego, object relations, and self experience come to be separable (though integrated) organizations of intrapsychic life and that we gain from seeing them that way. And second, that each is, in any event, present very early in life and has its own lines of development (see chapter 4).

Though I have referred to various theorists in developing my points along the way, I have stated that I am specifically not adopting any extant theoretical system. It is the perspective, the standpoint, embedded in these several psychologies, and the varying phenomena to which they address themselves, with which I shall work. Thus, for example, while I appreciate Fairbairn's (1941) argument that drives are object seeking and not only pleasure seeking and while I use his term *object relations theory*, in no other way will I make use of his overall theoretical system here. And while I have learned to recognize the clinical phenomena to which Kohut (1971, 1977) has called our attention, it is not his Self Psychology as a system to which I refer when I write of the perspective of self experience. And similarly, the view that I shall develop later on of central motives in human behavior diverges from Freud's (1905, 1920a) drive psychology; and my view of the perspective of the psychology of the ego, heavily influenced by my interest in ego defect from a developmental standpoint, is certainly not coterminous with ego psychology as developed by Freud (1923), A. Freud (1936), and Hartmann (1939). I do not specifically reject any of these theoretical conceptions, but they are not necessary for me to deal with in the task that I have set myself.

That task is the description of (1) the development of motivation and psychological organization in respect to the personal psychologies of drive, ego, object relations, and self experience and of (2) the clinical utility of working with these same four psychologies. These personal psychologies, in contrast to the theoretical ones, are formed in differentially significant moments of experience that have quite different shape and that are laid down as affectively charged active memory organizations of varied quality—now in terms of an experience of urge, now of achievement, coping, or mastery, now of object connection, now of self experience. These inevitably grow, for good or for ill, successfully or faultily, out of unavoidable experiences of childhood, given the inherent characteristics of human thought and feeling, and are part of every individual. As I shall discuss in chapter 6, in the course of development these different experiences are repeated again and again in different contexts with differing outcomes, gradually becoming interconnected with one another, so that eventually every psychic act potentially relates to all of these subjective experiences and comes to have multiple functions in relation to them. Thus the *phenomena* addressed by these several psychologies and all of our theories have central affective significance in the lives of individuals and therefore must be addressed clinically whatever the status of any particular *theoretical* formulation.

The question often comes up whether the four psychologies are best seen as truly *separate* psychologies or as differing *perspectives* on the phenomena. Though I prefer to reserve the full discussion of this for later on (chapters 5 and 6), I will state that I believe there is a basis in the development of the individual for thinking of them in both ways. Early on there are moments in the life of the infant where one or another psychology dominates experience (Pine, 1985) and, later on, some individuals achieve personalities organized primarily in one or another way; in these senses the four are separate psychologies. But there is also no doubt that in numerous less extreme instances of human psychic functioning, the four are blended and are best seen as alternative perspectives on experience. As perspectives, they can each be brought to bear on the description of any psychological experience. Much in the fashion of the proposal by Rapaport and Gill (1959) that a full accounting of any psychological event requires that it be described from each of five metapsychological points of view (economic, dynamic, structural, adaptive, genetic), I would here propose that any behavior can be described from four functional points of view: that is, in relation to drive gratification, ego function, object relations, and self experience. However, while as perspectives on experience each of the four can always in principle be brought to bear on the analysis of any psychic event, as truly separate psychologies one or another may be more frequently central. In my own clinical experience as I understand it at this point, issues of conflict over drive and its vicissitudes, of defense, and of the repetition of old internalized object relations seem to come up most often and seem most often to be clarifying when interpreted. Nonetheless, issues involved, say, in failures in boundary formation of the self or of ego defect, while coming up less often, seem absolutely crucial to recognize and deal with in those not infrequently seen individuals for whom they are central.

CHAPTER 3

The Four Psychologies in Clinical Work

I HAVE ALREADY suggested that I believe that many or most analysts in fact draw upon multiple perspectives in their day-to-day clinical work, without paying particular heed to the crossing of lines between conceptual models. Clinical work demands such breadth, lest patients be forced into narrower molds. In this chapter, I attempt to make some of these variations in clinical work explicit, first, by a discussion of the subject of "evenly suspended attention" (Freud, 1912) and, second, by a discussion of the special requirements of tact, phrasing, dosage, and timing as the scope of patients worked with analytically widens (Stone, 1954).

EVENLY SUSPENDED ATTENTION

Psychoanalytic technique proper came into being when Freud gave up forced association techniques and hypnosis and substituted open-ended listening, listening with evenly suspended attention to the content of the patient's associations. Provided that we listen with evenly hovering attention, uncommitted to any specific expectations regarding what is going on in a particular treatment hour, waiting to allow the clinical material to take whatever unique shape it will, we are constantly surprised—delightedly and profoundly—by the seemingly endless variability in the functioning of the human mind. But in spite of these continually renewed lessons of the indispensability of openmindedness, strong counterpressures work within us in the opposite direction. It is the natural tendency of mind to make sense of things, to make order out of disorder, to seek closure and certainty. Sitting with a patient, listening to the often mystifying flow of associations, the treating clinician's mind will quite naturally "find" ordering principles, "red threads" weaving through the content, "meanings."

Indeed we count on this tendency of mind in our clinical work. Freud's guideline of evenly hovering attention for the listening clinician makes sense only if we recognize its counterpart: the sense-making, meaning-finding, ordering tendencies of the human mind. Freud's idea was, of course, to allow meaning to emerge rather than to be imposed by preformed notions. The clinician's mind is never blank. It is filled with personal history, one's own analysis, the general background of what has been learned from all previous patients, the prior clinical history with a particular patient, and general theory. The intent of evenly hovering attention is to produce not blank minds, but uncommitted ones—minds receptive to the organization of this particular content from this particular patient in this particular hour in ways true to its potentially unique offering.

Total uncommittedness is an impossibility, and the first source of the interruption of evenly hovering attention is Freud's monumental theoretical achievement itself. For the creation of psychoanalytic theory, with its view of human functioning as organized around drives and conflict, itself creates basic expectations and assumptions about the potential meanings of the contents of an analytic hour. Thus, while we may approximate evenly hovering attention—that is, uncommitted listening—in relation to the particular contents of a particular hour, ordinarily we have in mind a general set of theoretical constructs that dictate what the *potential* meanings are in what we are hearing. Uncommitted listening to this particular hour generally occurs in the context of broader theoretical commitments regarding conceptions of personality development, personality organization, and their unfolding in the treatment situation. This is a profound limitation on truly evenhanded or uncommitted listening.

To highlight this issue in another way, let me overstate a certain paradox. As scientists, psychoanalytic clinicians work under a self-expectation to be true to the phenomena, to be servants to the data, to be reporters of the observed. This presses in the direction of openmindedness. But as professionals, psychoanalytic clinicians work under a self-expectation to be knowledgeable, to be expert in a body of knowledge which they can apply in the amelioration of psychic distress. Patients come to us, and pay us, to be experts, not scientists. This presses in the direction of closure.

To date, and not without struggle, psychoanalysis has produced, out of the tension between openmindedness and closure, the four psychologies that I have already outlined—ways of ordering the data of lives. These have evolved from the listening process—one or another analyst selectively attuned to one or another aspect of clinical phenomena. Though evenly hovering attention means that we hold all of this to the side as we allow the red threads of particular hours to show through, theoretical commitments, taken-for-granted views regarding development and pathology, can profoundly dictate the range of potential meanings to which we are receptive. Tendencies to organize the material along lines of conflict, of narcissistic transferences, of oedipal pathology, or of preoedipal pathology flow from theoretical commitments and not only from open-ended listening. Different theories lead us to approach the clinical hour with different questions in mind. And these can affect what we come to understand, how we phrase interpretations, and ultimately, therefore, both the entire conduct and presumably the outcome of an analysis.

These theory-derived questions are numerous. And I believe they are productive, not restrictive, when they are held in back of our minds—as *potential* ways of thinking of the associative content and its accompanying affect. The task of analytic listening remains that of suspension between knowledge of human functioning and open-ended ignorance of how a particular hour in a particular patient will come to be best understood.

The drive psychology, as analysts have worked with it since its beginnings with Freud, alerts us always to ask (silently, in nonverbalized ways even to ourselves, but always in the background, guiding our listening): what wish is being expressed? what is the relation of the wish to consciousness? what is the fantasy? and how does it reflect a compromise among wish and defense and reality? how is the wish being defended against? and how effective/ adaptive is the defense? can the particular anxiety seen be traced to this or that wish, ineffectively defended against? and can the particular guilt seen be understood in terms of the operation of conscience in relation to this or that wish? And similarly for symptoms and inhibitions: how do they reflect compromise formations among wish and defense and conscience and the patient's historical realities? And likewise for character: how have particular urges been transformed and meshed with defensive styles so as to contribute to characteristic and ordinarily ego syntonic modes of function? And related questions influence our historical/reconstructive/formulative view: what early under- or overgratifications of particular drives (and their related wishes) have occurred, producing early fixations and tendencies to regression? and is there any evidence for genetically greater drive strength in one or another area? or for early trauma that provoked increased activity around particular drives? Each of these genetic or traumatic factors can help account for resistance to change.

Quite familiar interpretations flow from such questions within the drive psychology. Thus, "So we can see that when you make a mess of your life and of your analysis, you're telling your mother, and me, that we can't make you be neat and clean—and though you're ashamed of the mess, you get too much pleasure from it to let it change." Or "When you speak to me about these intimate things it feels like you're secretly exhibiting yourself to your father once again, and you get so excited that you can no longer speak." Or "How comforting it is to believe that I am trying to get you to stop masturbating, against your wishes, so that you don't have to have the experience that you yourself want to stop but also feel that you are unable to." Or "Your rage at me feels safe to you; as long as we seem to be fighting, neither of us will know how arousing it is for you not only to fight but even to be here in the first place."

The questions from the drive psychology also apply powerfully to Freud's defining features of psychoanalysis—that is, transference and resistance. For the transference is understood ultimately in terms of the press of drives for satisfaction, now playing themselves out on the person of the analyst. And resistance is understood in terms of the automatic, unconsciously working counterpressures against the entry of conflictual drive derivatives into consciousness. So the questions: which drive? and how is it defended against? apply here as well.

The array of questions is long, and years of psychoanalytic work have demonstrated their fruitfulness. In classical psychoanalytic theory, the sexual urges (in their broad sense, as expanded by Freud) have remained first in importance in formulations regarding human drives, with aggression being a major second. And the questions, those listed and other related ones that could be added, seem at times (and in some patients) to provide us with entry into all we need to know about the person with whom we are working.

But is this really so? Is it true that such questions lead us to all we now know and need to know about human function? Of course not. I doubt that any clinical psychoanalysis is fully organized around conceptions of drives and their workings. Among drive theorists (historically and to some degree still) there is a tendency to formulate published cases in these terms, and this probably accurately represents much of the work, but such formulations reflect partially the available conceptual tools and partially social convention and social conformity pressure among analysts. Clearly other questions, stemming from different theoretical bases, can be formulated.

Some of those deriving from the psychology of the ego, particularly those related to defense, seem almost indistinguishable from some of those from the psychology of drive—being the other side of the same coin. Thus, we can ask: what defenses are operative against the drives? and how effective (rigid, flexible, reliably available or not) are they? But even here the questions extend beyond the drive psychology: how are affects being defended against (A. Freud, 1936)? and how is relatedness itself being defended against (Modell, 1984)? The examples of drive-linked interpretation that I gave by and large include reference to defense as well as to the urge being defended against. Other interpretations more fully in the domain of defense may, for example, take the form: "As long as you won't allow me to matter to you in the least, you can go on feeling that there is no reason to tell me anything that may be upsetting to you." Or "Your chronic alertness and reserve serve to nip any emotion in the bud; you certainly won't be angry, or sad, or excited—that would be too dangerously unpredictable." Or "As long as you can feel convinced that you know what I'm going to say even before I say it, you can feel there is no reason to listen to me in the first place, and you can ride right over my words."

But the questions stimulated by our psychology of the ego, and particularly of its development, go well beyond questions of defense. They include a whole set of questions of the kind: what tools of adaptation have failed to develop or have developed aberrantly?—for example, tension maintenance? the capacity for delay? object constancy? concern for others? the socialization of urge? The list could go on and on. Interpretations here include: "Because you never felt you had a picture of a good parent to hold in mind as a child, my going away is especially hard for you; you can't even let yourself anticipate it." Or "You're so convinced that once again you won't be able to stop the anxiety from flooding you that you get anxious even before it starts, so to speak, and can't do the things that you've learned help you maintain some control." Or "The sense of shame that you feel seems to come largely from the belief that you're defective—that you can't control any of your urges."

Within recent analytic writings such issues have been subsumed within the larger question: to what degree do we think of psychic function in terms of defect (or deficit) or in terms of conflict? The question, largely stimulated by Kohut's (1977) formulations regarding deficits in early selfobject relationships which produce deficiencies in the self experience, but also an outgrowth of a developmental point of view, is too either/or and too bounded by experience with analyzable (even marginally analyzable) patients. Certainly when we recognize that the infant is not born with his or her adult tools for adaptation fully in place, we also recognize that they have to develop—and therefore can develop poorly or well, whether or not they are also involved in and even stunted as a result of conflict. And psychoanalysis as a general psychology has to recognize pathology beyond the range of the analyzable, and there concepts of defect in ego function are indispensable and unavoidable. But I believe such questions to be relevant to most analyses as well, to varying degrees (and see chapter 10).

The psychology of object relations produces yet other questions to ask of the clinical data, yet other perspectives on the history of the individual and the workings of pathology. Object relations theory is not a single theory, and the questions within these theories that I find most useful, sitting somewhere in the back of my mind as I do clinical work, include: what old object relationship is being repeated? and which of the roles in the object relationship is the subject (the patient) enacting—his own or that of the other? or both? Is the patient behaving like the person he was? he wished to be in the parents' eyes? they wanted him to be? they were? he wished they were? And what early passive experiences are being repeated actively? Such questions are based on the idea that all significant early relationships get repeated in action later on, either out of efforts to repeat pleasure experiences or to master traumatic ones. And the "pleasure experiences" obviously need not be "pleasurable" in "objective" terms (that is, you or I might not think of them as pleasurable); but they are the carriers of the relationship with the parents of childhood, and however good or bad those experiences may have been, they are experiences with the only parents the patient has had, and so reflect forms of attachment and familiarity, and thus safety, no matter what pain they may also include. Thus the questions can be reframed to ask such things as: do these behaviors repeat earlier experiences with the parents and thus serve to hold onto those relationships? or are they efforts to master old traumatizing relationships by repeating them actively with others? And then there are historically based questions: to what degree are these relations as carried in memory, enacted in identification, or repeated in action—to what degree are they veridical renditions of what happened in childhood? Presumably they are never fully veridical and, in any event, we will never really know (see Spence, 1982), but (and here the drive and ego psychologies interweave with that of object relations) they presumably reflect the *experienced* object relation, that experience determined by the drive state or ego state of the subject at the moment of the relational event. Thus, once again, it is *that* experience that is laid down as memory, not anything that can be called an objective event in its own right. There is no objective event in this sense, only subjective experience; and yet the sorting out of personal history, of its realities and its subjectivities, can, I believe, be exceptionally useful to the patient in analysis.

Interpretations in relation to internalized object relations are certainly common. Thus, "Yes, your parents seemed to be cruel to you, but they were the only parents you had and so you keep them with you through continued cruelty to me and to others." Or "Everybody, myself included, becomes your father in your mind's eye, and then you know just how to behave—as his naive and innocent little seductress." Or "The pain of the abandonment you felt was so great that you continually try to free yourself of it by inflicting it on others." Or "You were so enraged at your mother for so obviously being your father's only interest that there was no other way you could remember her but as retaliatory and herself enraged at you." Though some of these statements include implicit reference to wishes, they are phrased primarily in terms of the dynamics of continuance, repetition, and attempted mastery of internal dramas, derived from history in some way, and carried inside.

And last to questions for the clinical situation stimulated by a psychology of self experience. As noted already, I am here neither subscribing to nor rejecting the specific formulations advanced by Kohut (1977) and others under the name Self Psychology, but rather referring to a range of features of the human situation variously addressed by different contributors. Among the questions that I find useful (again as questions sitting in the back of my mind—that is, as potential modes of conceptualizing the clinical data or addressing the actual patient) are those having to do with boundaries, integration, and esteem: how stable a sense of differentiated self boundaries is present? or how much are fantasies of merger, enactments of merger, or panics regarding loss of boundaries a factor in the clinical situation? how do the differentiated boundaries stand up in relation to the stresses of living? how much is derealization or depersonalization a part of the picture? And also: how much is discontinuity of the self experience present? does it feel subjectively (to the analyst) that one is with the same patient each session or is there a subjective sense of discontinuity? And how much does the patient experience himself or herself as the center of action in his or her own life? as the "cause" of that life? And further: what is the ongoing sense of self-value, of esteem? and what pathological efforts to right imbalances in that subjective state of self are present: grandiosity? denial? flights into activity? disdain of others?

Interpretations here may take many forms: "You got frightened just now when I used the word *we* because it made you feel I was invading you, just as it used to feel with your mother." Or "Succeeding at school made you feel like a person, separate from others, so you rushed back into failure to get your parents and me reinvolved with you." Or "Your anger at me and others is a comfort to you; it makes you feel filled, like you know who you are, that I can't take you over." Or "Your experience of not being responded to by your parents made you feel that you lost touch with who you were, and so when I don't greet you sufficiently as you come in you can't believe that you and I are the same two people who worked together yesterday." Or "You're showing me what your parents thought of themselves and of you by acting in such a way as to advertise how worthless you are." Or "You've never felt that you're having your own life—but rather only the one you are living for your father—and so when the idea of changing comes up, it only seems to mean living a different life for *me*."

Each of the four psychologies has a somewhat different conception of humankind and our essential tasks. Drive psychology emphasizes the taming, socialization, and gratification of drives. Ego psychology emphasizes the development of defense with respect to the internal world, adaptation with respect to the external world, and reality testing with respect to both. Object relations theory focuses on the task of simultaneously carrying within us (through identification and internalized object relations) the record of the history of our significant relationships—which is essential to our humanness and is a basis for social living—and, on the other hand, of freeing ourselves from the absolute constraints of those relationships so that new experiences can be greeted, within limits, as new and responded to on their own, contemporary, terms. And psychologies of the self focus on the diverse tasks of forming a differentiated and whole sense of self (both in contradistinction to and in relation to the other), of establishing the self as a center of initiative and as the owner of one's inner life, and of developing an ongoing sense of subjective worth. Evenly hovering attention will be most evenhanded when attention allows for the organization of the session content in these diverse ways.

THE QUESTION OF VARIATION IN TECHNIQUE

Certainly variations in clinical technique are part of most analyses at some times. In Eissler's (1953) paper in which he introduces the notion of (subsequently analyzable) parameters he gives official recognition to what was, in any event, an unofficial fact of clinical life—namely, that many an analysis requires a modification in technique at some point. The concept of parameters legitimized this, as it were. Those of us who supervise analysts in training can all point to instances where the trainee was so excessively scrupulous about adhering to "standard" technique as to make a mockery of it.

In fact, variations in technique may be so regularly present (at *occasional moments*) in analyses as to make it more appropriate to think of technique in terms of theme and variations rather than in any more monolithic way. There is no doubt in my mind that clinical experience teaches that quiet listening in the context of evenly hovering attention and of the triad of neutrality, relative anonymity, and nongratification of drive aims (abstinence), coupled with interventions of an interpretive sort especially attuned to resistance and transference, is not only the most cautious but an immensely productive way to work. That is the theme. I shall not try to catalogue the variations in any general sense. One person's variation is often another's standard way of working—for example, occasional congratulations after some major life event, giving information (for example, a referral or consultation name for a family member or friend) when the patient asks for it, acknowledging a bit of tactlessness in our own work. Even to mention these requires my adding that none of these need be either/or—that is, acting but not analyzing; they can include both.

But my main point is that work with the substantive content and intrapsychic processes varyingly addressed by each of the four psychologies is not a variation in technique but rather, I believe, common to the work of most of us. I raise this whole issue because, as I have discussed these ideas previously, I have been confronted with the challenge that "you cannot work in four different ways." Usually, I think, that challenge (in our current climate) comes from the idea that any mention of self means one is working in the manner that has evolved within Kohut's Self Psychology (see Goldberg, 1978), and that therefore I must be espousing markedly different modes of working—perhaps only two ways, perhaps four. Quite the contrary; I believe that there is nothing in the material I have presented thus far that requires any automatic variations in technique. What varies is the substantive content that is addressed by interpretation, and to some extent, perhaps, the intrapsychic processes or "mechanisms" described in interpretations, but not the main theme of technique as I have described it.

I have occasionally been asked how I decide which of the four psychologies to apply in a particular session, as though that, too, represented some arbitrary variation in technique. But my answer is straightforward: I do not "apply" anything. I listen with evenly hovering attention until I feel I understand something, and something that it makes sense to say in this particular session. The critical point is that what I understand may be in the terms of the substantive content and mechanisms highlighted by any of the several psychologies. But listening and understanding remain the keys. This answer is no different from the answer to the question, how do you decide whether to address the oedipal or preoedipal material? the maternal or paternal aspects of the transference? or whether to interpret in the transference or outside of it? We can probably outline a rough clinical guideline or two, but mostly we listen, try to understand where the "point of urgency" (Strachey,

1934) is now in this session, and respond based on that understanding. So, too, with the material of the four psychologies.

On the other hand, if one holds in mind the kinds of questions and issues that flow from each of the several psychologies, I believe analysts will find themselves thinking about clinical material in more diverse ways. In this sense, ideas stemming from the several psychologies can "lead" and not only "follow" the material—that is, they can provide us with other ways to think about it. Thus, while, from a drive point of view, we can hear a preoccupation with a particular form of satisfaction in terms of a conflicted wish that neither allows satisfaction nor allows the patient to move beyond it, we can also, from other points of view and at other times (or in other patients), hear it as a preoccupation that stems from the patient's fear that he or she will not be able to retain control over the impulse unless it is always kept in mind (defense); or as an identification with a parental style of thinking, an identification that holds the lost object near (object relational); or as a preoccupation with a wished-for pleasure that is serving primarily to ward off awareness of an empty inner experience (self experience).

All of this leads me to restate that, while the psychoanalytic narratives constructed with a patient are potentially wide ranging (Schafer, 1983), they are not conceptually without limit. I believe that the concepts and the languages of the several psychologies addressed here are likely to subsume the range of these narratives, though, of course, there are infinite individual variations within each as well. All individuals have experiences of many shapes and the multiple perspectives of the several psychologies are well suited to address them all, and certainly better suited to do so than any one alone.

But there *is* a significant technical variation that I wish to address and that I think has an important place in psychoanalytic work. That has to do with those aspects of tact, timing, and phrasing that are drawn upon in recognition of and respect to momentary or more broad-based fragility of a particular patient. In general, these modifications have to do with increasing the "holding" (Winnicott, 1963b) aspects of the analytic situation. Modell (1984), drawing on Winnicott's concept, has described the holding aspects of the analytic situation as it is ordinarily carried out, apart from any variations in technique; by this he refers to such things as the analyst's reliability, nonretaliation, being there for the patient's needs, and having a better grasp of the patient's psychic life than does the patient (p. 91). Loewald (1960) advances a similar argument, though without reference to holding per se, in his recognition of the implicit mother-child aspects of the transference situation which make reintegration possible following the analytically wrought mini-disintegrations.

Others, however, have offered technical modifications to increase these holding aspects in situations of particular need. Thus, Mark Grunes (1984) described such issues with respect to questions of "dosage" with difficult patients, that is, the recognition of and adjustment to what the patient can tolerate taking in at any particular time. Winnicott (1963b) himself, in distinguishing between abstinence in respect to drive aims and, on the other hand, possible gratification of ego needs, expands on what is in effect a further holding aspect of analytic technique. Arnold Modell (1984), also, contrasts the background status of the holding function in the so-called classical case with its greater centrality in cases involving developmental arrest. And I (Pine, 1984) discussed these holding considerations as well as other more explicit alterations in the phrasing and timing of interpretation in work with more consistently fragile and generally unanalyzable patients; these alterations are all matters of the analyst's style of verbalization and do not include more active supportive measures (Werman, 1984). But they do meet object or ego needs without gratifying drive aims for the most part. In fact, however, the need for such variations on a momentary basis may come up in any analysis, say early on when an anxiety-ridden patient is first beginning work on the couch, or at later phases when particularly difficult material of the patient's past life and current functioning is at center stage. But, it seems clear to me, the aim of such variations—that is, of explicitly increasing the holding or safety features* of the analytic situation—is to make the regular work of analysis, carried on in the usual way, possible. That is, by aiding some patients over particular rough spots at moments, it makes possible a relatively standard analysis, centered on interpretation, neutrality, abstinence, and anonymity.

This whole question is sometimes referred to, generally not convincingly, I feel, in terms that suggest that a patient was given a period of "psychotherapy" before the "psychoanalysis proper" could begin. But it seems to me that that is more verbal gymnastics than convincing clinical sense, designed to separate the "copper" of psychotherapy from the "pure gold" (Freud, 1919) of analysis. I believe that the picture of occasional and momentary variations in technique during the course of what is essentially an analysis

---

*I hesitate to use the word *supportive* because that calls to mind a whole different approach to treatment that I am not referring to (see Werman, 1984).

better describes the process than some seemingly clear division between the psychotherapeutic and the psychoanalytic phases of the same treatment. (This is not meant to suggest that some patients in analytic psychotherapy do not later decide to undertake an analysis, but that is a whole different issue from the one of modifications in technique based on psychological need.)

Though in an earlier paper (Pine, 1984) I discussed such variations in technique loosely with respect to "fragile" patients, and later (1988) more specifically as applied to the pathology of defect in ego function or of deficits in parental handling, in fact I do not believe that such modifications, when necessary, are tied solely to the issues of any one or two of the four psychologies. Clinical and historical contexts in particular patients can readily make it such that a technical modification (a parameter), or rather, particular attention to the holding features of the analytic situation, may become necessary with respect to any or all of the kinds of intrapsychic issues I have been discussing, a modification that makes the continuance of the analysis (or even the *onset* of an analysis) possible. Primitive drive issues or particularly painful, overwhelming, or humiliating object-relational issues—as much as ego defect and self deficit issues—may at times require those special modifications of tact, timing, and dosage that broadly go under the rubric holding. Awareness of this, in my experience, increases the range and number of those patients who can be worked with analytically.

CHAPTER 4

The Four Psychologies in the Developmental Process

IN THE PREVIOUS chapter I attempted to demonstrate that it is useful, clinically, to think in terms of the four psychologies. In parallel form in this chapter I hope to show that it is plausible, developmentally, to think similarly. While I believe that especially significant developments take place in respect to each of the psychologies very early on, I shall argue that significant developments take place in each through the life cycle as well.

Mitchell (1984), in arguing for the full life-cycle relevance of object relations as a basic organizer of human development and functioning, uses the metaphor of a "developmental tilt" to show the markedly different way in which object relations are ordinarily accommodated to the classical drive/conflict theory as he sees it. He writes:

One of the most important devices through which accommodation has been accomplished, leading to pervasive implications in the way object relations concepts have been shaped, has been the "developmental tilt"—i.e., Freud was correct in understanding the mind in terms of conflicts among drives; object relations are also important, but *earlier*. For many strategists of accommodation the pillar of classical metapsychology, the structural model, is understood to provide an adequate framework for an account of human experience, both normal and pathological, and that account depicts the conflict among various drive derivatives, and between drive derivatives and defensive functions of the ego and the superego. When a theorist following this strategy wants to introduce various relational needs and processes as primary in their own right, as irreducible, as neither merely gratifiers nor defenders against drives, they are often introduced as operative before the tripartite structures of id, ego, and superego have become separated and articulated. Theories concerned with linear continuity necessarily present the classical theory of neurosis as centered around sexual and aggressive conflicts at the oedipal phase. They set object relations formulations into pre-existing theory by arguing that they pertain to a developmental epoch prior to the differentiation of psychic structure in the earliest relationship of the mother and infant. The traditional model is jacked up, and new relational concepts are slid in underneath. [In an] architectural metaphor, it is as if a new, complex, and roomy foundation level has been set underneath an older edifice; the upper stories remain just as they were, but the center of gravity has shifted downward. The original structure is intact but unoccupied; the scene of the action has moved downward to the lower levels. (pp. 476–477)

Mitchell then goes on to discuss various theorists from this standpoint, and summarizes:

Each of these theorists—Klein, Balint, Winnicott, Mahler, and Kohut—maintains a loyalty, in one form or another, to classical drive theory. One (Mahler) maintains the earlier model in its essentials; another (Klein) preserves its language while changing its meanings; another (Winnicott) proclaims his loyalty although the original model no longer figures meaningfully in his formulations. Despite this diversity in degrees of fealty, each author requires accommodation to make room for his or her own contribution, and therefore many of these innovations have been introduced into psychoanalytic theory via the developmental tilt; consequently the dynamic issues they depict tend to get characterized as infantile, pre-oedipal, immature, and their persistence in later life is often regarded as a residue of infantilism, rather than as an expression of human relational needs extending throughout the life cycle. (p. 478)

Mitchell's characterization of the "developmental tilt" in the literature could be extended in substantially similar form to the way issues of self and of ego development are sometimes viewed as well; and I shall argue for the full life-cycle relevance of each of them. While an argument can be made in some clinical instances that failures in *early* ego organization, self differentiation, and/or core attachment to significant objects take a certain precedence in the organization of the personality and in the forms of psychopathology ever after, the reverse is not true. That is, it is not the case that, if the relevant ego/self/object developments take place adequately early on, they are no longer significant for later aspects of the developmental process, of the organization of the personality, or of the forms of psychopathology.

There is always a danger of caricature when one states what the so-called pure classical drive theorist would say about thus and so. In fact, however, I believe that most of the phenomena that I shall describe here are well known to all dynamically oriented developmental theorists and figure in the ongoing work of all analytic clinicians, whatever theory they espouse. But, consistent with the stance I have been taking throughout, I believe it is clarifying and broadening to view such phenomena nonreductionistically, from the standpoint of the four psychoanalytic psychologies.

Let me start with just one example of the conceptual slanting that can come from a view of development in the terms of only one of the psychologies. The concept of latency is one that has a firm place within psychoanalytic developmental theory. It gives name to that period of childhood when the individual is in school, away from the intensity of bodily and relational linkage to the primary love objects of childhood (in contrast to the preschooler at home with mother), and not yet subject to the biologically induced storms triggered by puberty. The concept of latency signifies that no new major drive aims (such as orality, anality, oedipal wishes, and, later, adolescent sexuality) emerge during this period; that considerable repression and aim inhibition take place vis-à-vis the urges of the period of infantile sexuality; that residual toned-down sexual interests can be displaced, outside the home, to teachers and peers; and that the major new learnings that take place are less involved with the body than they were in the earliest years (feeding, toileting, self care) or will be in adolescence (with the "learnings" regarding the *sexual* body).

But latency is a concept that has its meaning primarily within the drive psychology. There is nothing "latent" in the period, say, ages six or seven to eleven or twelve, with regard to developments in the spheres of ego, self, or object relations. It is well known that this period is a major time of ego development, both with respect to the consolidation of intrapsychic defense and with respect to the mastery of reality and expansion of adaptation that is seen in school learning and the extension of relations beyond the home to the peer group. Similarly, while there are of course forerunners, highly significant developments in self-esteem, in the sense of personal worth vis-à-vis others, take shape in this period around experiences with peers and with success or failure in school learning. The glories and humiliations dating from this childhood period, and affecting self-esteem, are much represented in the memories and affect life of patients in psychoanalysis. The fact that such memories may derive some of their meaning from yet earlier ones already carried in memory in no way eliminates the shaping potential of new tasks, opportunities, and failures. And, last, object relations: here, too, this is not a period of latency. Rather, many of the internalized object relations that are repetitively reenacted later in life appear to date from this mid-childhood period—from the way one experienced oneself as treated by either parent (or siblings) and the way one experienced the parents as treating each other. Thus latency, a concept within the drive psychology, should not be mistaken as a time of latency in respect to ego, self, and object relations developments. As in this example, we will get our fullest picture of clinically relevant developmental events by looking at phenomena in terms of each of the four psychologies.

SOME INTRODUCTORY CONCEPTS

Earlier (Pine, 1981, 1985), I advanced the idea that intrapsychic life is organized differently at different moments; and I used this idea as a way of encompassing the wide range of phenomena addressed by the four psychologies. Thus, there are times in the infant's day when the press of hunger or, soon after, the cry for the breast or bottle when hungry (based on the memory of previous gratifications) is the central focus of psychological experience. Though such a moment can be of great significance, however, it does not preclude the equally great significance of other moments, quite differently focused. Thus, that same infant, at another time, will be caught up in the exercise of eye-hand coordination, reaching for a familiar crib object, gurgling with glee at the mastery of grasping. As the first of these moments is central to a drive psychology, the second is central to an aspect of an ego psychology—the exercise of ego apparatuses in the service of adaptation or mastery. And yet again another moment: this time we imagine the infant placed in her crib by her mother, who then departs, and the infant easing into sleep, or uneasily cranky, or crying vigorously, and the mother returning or not, using voice, or physical contact, and varied affective responses to the infant—all of which presumably lead to a laying down in the infant of one or another object-related image, images of self and other in relation, images that color subsequent relations and expectations in the face of separation or connection or control or autonomy—all building blocks of a psychology of internalized object relations (Kernberg, 1976). And consider as a last example, the moment of an infant's melting into her mother's breast as she falls asleep after nursing, or wakeful and exploring her mother's face with hand and eye—moments that have been seen (Mahler et al., 1975; Pine, 1986b) as central, respectively, to the infant's experience of merger or of beginning differentiation, aspects of what I have been referring to as the psychology of self experience.

The point is that one does not have to make a choice among competing postulated (or witnessed) experiences in the life of a child as to their developmental impact. Or, at least, one does not have to make such a choice on *temporal* grounds. In different moments, there is time for all of them; no single moment tells us what the infant is "really" like. Of course, one may make a choice among such moments in terms of their affective and developmental significance, and may construct one or another theory of personality and development based upon the centrality accorded to these, or like, or other such moments. But I contend that each of these moments, and innumerable others, differently organized, have major affective and developmentally formative significance, and that our theories would do well to encompass them all.

By the word *moments*, I am not referring to a literal moment or to any 'particular temporal duration. A moment, rather, can be extended over time or brief, can be once in a while or recurrent. I refer to periods of time, however long, when experience is organized primarily in "this" way rather than in "that" way—and later more in "that" way than "this." But in moments, thus defined, we can find a place for the developmental significance of the many and varied phenomena addressed by the several psychologies of drive, ego, object relations, and self.

Further, I am not arguing for the exclusivity of such moments, as though one or another is the possession of one or another of the psychologies. For, though at times it is useful to think of such moments as primarily organized in one or another way, it is also possible to bring the perspective of each of the psychologies to bear on any one of them and to see their relevance in turn for the issues addressed by each psychology. Thus, in the instance of the hungry infant crying for breast or bottle, given above to illustrate phenomena addressed by a psychology of drive, we can readily recognize that object images are also being laid down in memory during the experience, that repeated experiences of gratification, or of an unresponsive (say, depressed) feeder (mother) will come to affect the infant's self state and its affective tone; and from yet another perspective the infant's capacity for delay in the face of hunger, or say, for a differentiated call to the mother, are indications of developing defensive and adaptive (ego) capacities. So, too, for all of the other examples used—they are not solely formative for the issues of the psychology for which I used them as exemplars. The infant grasping a toy may pull it to her mouth for substitutive sucking (*drive*) or hold it near as a transitional-like *object relation*, connected to the mother; and, in the grasping, mastery of such things as eye-hand coordination (*ego*) are also bedrocks of *self-esteem* (White, 1963; Broucek, 1979; Pine, 1982). As mental life expands, and wish and fantasy and cognitive elaborations of every variety take on a fuller role, then any behavioral event will be endowed with all of the psychological meaning that any particular individual brings to it, meanings addressed by each of the four psychologies.

I would like to introduce one other forerunner idea before embarking on a fuller description of the developmental process in terms of the four psychologies. That has to do with the role of inputs from the surround.

The formed adult person is pretty much a self-causing system. That is, while we are certainly influenced by inputs from our surround, what we elicit from that surround, and what "appeals" to us in it and is therefore selected by us (Pine, 1982), and the environment that we choose and create for ourselves altogether, are very much influenced by who we are, by our central motives and mechanisms. This is never completely the case—since life's opportunities and accidents affect us all—and it is probably less the case in earlier and yet earlier childhood. The child and, before that, the infant, are certainly much more at the mercy of inputs from the surround— negative or positive, absences or presences.

But there, too, the infant or child is not a purely reactive system, not passive in the face of experience. It was Freud's great achievement to bring internal causation into the infant psychological system—in the form of the biologically based and epigenetically programmed drives. There is more to this of course. Hartmann (1939) added the recognition of the inborn ego apparatuses and infant researchers (for example, Escalona, 1963; Sander, 1977) have shown the active role of the infant in the mother-infant dyad— but it is not relevant for me to enlarge upon this here.

Rather, I wish to contrast Freud's drive theory to Kohut's (1977) Self Psychology, wherein external causation plays a much larger role. It is well known that Kohut's espousal of a view that readily leads to a good-parent/ bad-parent picture of development, which is then corrected in the mirroring or idealizing relation to the analyst, is one of the points of radical disjunction from the classical drive theory. But other theorists who observe infants have also, inevitably, given recognition to the role of the parents in shaping the child. Winnicott recognizes the "environmental provision" and the "facilitating environment" (1965), and Mahler et al. (1975) certainly see the two-way street of mother-infant interaction culminating in separation-individuation. Kohut is taken to task more, by traditionalists at least, because of the relative exclusivity of his view and because he sometimes appears to have built so much of his treatment technique around it. But, and here is my main point, there is no way we can ignore the role of inputs from the surround in relation to the development of the phenomena addressed by *each* of the psychologies and by no means only in relation to the "self" of Kohut's Self Psychology.

In introducing the concept of the "average expectable environment," Hartmann (1939) said, in effect, that the environment is of indispensable significance for development but that, for now, as a theoretical convenience, we will not focus on it but rather will assume it to be "average," that is, adequate for development to proceed. And this was sufficient for Hartmann's purposes—to develop the place of adaptation in a psychology of drives. But, as clinicians, developmentalists, parents, and former children, we well know that it is the precise individual environment, and not the average expectable one, that matters in development. And therein lies a tale of facilitation, aberration, or obstruction vis-à-vis the phenomena addressed by *each* of the psychologies, and by no means only by a psychology of self experience.

Thus, we well know that seduction, overindulgence, or undergratification of drive aims can wreak havoc with the optimal course of the development of drives—their taming, socialization, and delay on the one hand; their integration, expression, and sublimation on the other. And developments in the ego sphere are profoundly affected by the demands placed upon the person—with stress beyond adapting to at one extreme and facilitation and stimulation to learning and adaptation at the other—as well as by the very functioning of the parents themselves, who inevitably, through identification, become models for defense, adaptation, and reality testing. And the object relations psychology as I am using it, the internalization and repetition of such relationships as experienced by the child, is by definition a compound of the actual behaviors of significant objects and the affect and drive state of the experiencing subject. And optimal praise, allowance of individuation, and again models for identification will profoundly affect developments in the spheres of esteem, differentiation of boundaries, and self experience altogether. So inputs from the surround have significant effects in the domains of each of the four psychologies.

With these preliminary comments in mind let us turn to the developmental array itself.

EARLY DEVELOPMENTS IN THE FOUR PSYCHOLOGIES

To argue that significant developments continue to occur throughout the life span in relation to phenomena addressed by each of the four psychologies, and thus to argue (along with Mitchell, 1984) against the developmental tilt, is *not* to say that early developments and later developments are equal in weight for the individual life. In what follows, I wish to argue against the developmental tilt (that other-than-drive issues matter early but then drop out as major independent factors in mental functioning), but not to fall so completely into a life-span view as to fail to recognize a special *formative* role for very early processes—and to recognize this in the domain of *each* of the four psychologies. With regard to the last point, in one or another view failures in early development are emphasized especially with respect to one or another set of phenomena: an integrated self with goals and ideals, or an intact ego, for example. But I believe that issues of core early structuralization, or internalization, or intrapsychic differentiation—in different areas— are essential in the domains of each of the four psychologies.

For these early developments, one can think in terms of the *creation* of an intrapsychic world. It is not that the infant is born with nothing "inside the mind"; Freud's "drives," Hartmann's "ego apparatuses," and recent infant researchers' descriptions of the adaptive and relational capacities of the infant all speak to biological endowment. But these inborn givens notwithstanding, considerable early developmental work must take place for the creation of an intrapsychic world such as is already evident in childhood and is seen in full array in the psychoanalysis of adults. This is a world of fantasies and wishes and preferred gratifications and taboos, of individually preferred modes of coping, of internalized object relations, and of some familiar ongoing sense of self. The role of inputs from the surround may be at its greatest in relation to these early developments, for, after the formation of a differentiated intrapsychic world, the individual is much more of that self-causing and self-sustaining system that I referred to earlier. That is, a being has emerged whose motives, cognitive contents, and functional processes are carried inside in a sustained way that makes for relative continuity of the life process—with inner-determined processes imposing themselves on the environment, selecting and eliciting, differentially, from that environment, and automatically and by no means always consciously charting a course through that environment.

Such crucial early developments in the sphere of the drive psychology have been referred to in numerous ways. Freud (1900), for example, wrote of the development of the "wish" as the linkage of a current tension state to the memory image of a previous satisfaction of that state; more broadly this involves the ways in which bodily urges get cognitive representation and become part of a wish/fantasy system of mind. Winnicott, pointing out that instinctual drives can be experienced as external to the "going on being" of an infant, like "a clap of thunder or a hit" (1960a, p. 141), implies an early developmental task in which the drives become *owned* by the individual, part of the "I," not later to be experienced in the form of "I don't know what came over me" or "I wasn't myself." And writers on the psychology of the borderline child (Rosenfeld and Sprince, 1963) noting an absence of the achievement of "phase dominance" regarding the drives (that is, an organization of urges such that one or another is central at one or another appropriate early developmental epoch—such as the oral, anal, and oedipal phases), imply a task of creating a hierarchy of drives—some internal ordering, specialization, "seniority" among them—at least at different times. And earlier (Pine, 1970), I endeavored to show how drive-defense relationships early on become structuralized, in the sense of long lasting and resistant to change, through the development of multiple function; that is, as these drive-defense relationships come to serve functions with regard to, say, gratification, object relationship, adaptation, and sense of self, they become more firmly anchored in the personality, difficult to dislodge. Each of these, and more, are part of what I refer to as the creation of an intrapsychic world in the domain of the drive psychology. Not only ownership, hierarchical organization, and the achievement of multiple function, but also the attachment of drive-linked wishes to objects in preferred modes of gratification, and some core socialization of urge—some bowing to the reality principle by the development of delay, aim inhibition, and defense altogether—are part of the early core achievements in the area of drives that are essential to our humanness and to optimal, or even just adequate, functioning later on.

There can certainly be failures in the attainment of these early achievements. In such instances we may see impulsive, violent, or otherwise destructive acting upon disowned urges as ownership, defense, and socialization processes fail to occur. Or we may see polymorphous perverse functioning in the face of failed hierarchical organization, or promiscuity and/or detachment in the face of failed attachment of drive-based wishes to objects, or panic and flooding in the face of faulty control processes. Each of these can, of course, come about by multiple routes. There is no one-to-one correspondence between developmental event and subsequent outcome, no way to read developmental history automatically from any surface behavioral manifestation (A. Freud, 1970). For example, it is clear that both promiscuity and detachment can be the resultant of either defensive avoidance or developmental failure of attachment. I only mean to suggest that all of these possibilities should be "dreamt of in our philosophy" and that one significant set of such possibilities has to do with early developments involving the core patterning, the structuralization and hierarchical organization, the socialization and integration of biologically based drives—or the failures in any of these.

As we turn to look at the early creation of an intrapsychic world, or, otherwise stated, the early structural/formative developments in the domain of ego, object relations, and self, it will be evident that the phenomena addressed are not always different from those discussed earlier with respect to drive—sometimes different, but not always. These are matters not only of additional phenomena of human function but also of altered perspective on any single phenomenon.

Let us turn now to some of the early developments in the domain addressed by a psychology of object relations. Here, too, there are various core developmental tasks. First is the establishment of a basic attachment to objects—in this case the primary caretaker. Built on a probable biologically based attachment (Bowlby, 1969), there nonetheless develops not only a specificity of attachment to a primary love object, but a quality of this attachment such that there can be some hope and expectation of comfort and gratification in the connection to the object. In patients deemed analyzable and thus selected for psychoanalysis, we can take this core attachment for granted—because its absence would have led to a decision against analyzability. Such a core relationship is the stage on which the action of an analysis takes place. With that stage in place, we can take it for granted and focus on the action (the meanings found in free association and transference); but without it, the action would not take place. In an earlier paper (Pine, 1986a; and see chapter 10), I tried to show how failures in such basic trust can lead to failures in the development from panic anxiety to signal anxiety and from indiscriminate need-satisfying relationships to specificity of attachment, and further to failures in the development of phase dominance of urges, of the taming of aggression, of the maturation of defense, and of the establishment of positive self-esteem.

In another early developmental aspect of object relations, Sandler and Rosenblatt (1962) show how the individual develops a "representational world." This is the means through which the world of internalized object relations gets recorded in memory and can, thenceforth, lead to expectations and actions that are determinative of later object relations, patterned on these early internal representations. The mind gets filled out (or filled up), so to speak, with the residues of early relationships as experienced, and this is a core part of that creation of an intrapsychic world that must take place early on. Nothing in human life is absolutely static, and it is of course the case that the representational world of internalized object relations can also undergo later modification. But, in the terms given us by Piaget (1952) for the description of continuity and change in mental life, once a representational world is established in reasonably articulated form—that is, once there is a set of expectations and response readinesses vis-à-vis objects and a conception of how self and other will mutually interact—later relationships are in substantial part *assimilated* to these beliefs and wishes, and only in part will new "real" events in the relational world lead to *accommodation* (alteration) in the inner representational world in response to these realities.

Failures in these basic developments in the object relations sphere would be equivalent in impact to those, above, in the drive sphere—powerfully, and negatively, affecting the subsequent life course. "Failure" regarding core object attachment and trust means just that, a minimal or unreliable development of those features. But there can be no "failure" of the development of a representational world in the same sense; *some* inner cognitive representation will develop (with the possible exception of autistic states). Here, *failure* can refer only to the development of an unremittingly destructive and nongratifying inner map of the experienced world.

Core early developments in the domain of self experience have also been addressed by numerous writers. At their center is the differentiation of the "I-you" boundary to begin with. Ideas in this domain are prominently connected with the work of Mahler (Mahler et al., 1975) and, earlier, of Spitz (1957); Mahler (1968), additionally, has written of gross failures of self-other differentiation in what she refers to as "symbiotic psychosis." The emergence of a self, both out of the affectively compelling moments of merger as the infant melts into the mother's breast after nursing (see chapter 11), and via the expansion of motility and affect which creates a sense of a self (through movement and affective fullness), is a central development of early childhood, strikingly notable when it is absent (Mahler, 1968; Pine, 1979b). Beyond this, another centerpiece of the self experience is what Winnicott (1960a) reaches for in his description of true self–false self experience. He writes of the infant's "spontaneous gesture" that, when met adequately by the world's response (in the form of the primary caretaker), can lead to a confirmation for the infant of the safety and fittedness of expressing his or her inner processes to and in that world—the beginnings of a "true self." It is, actually, a simple conditioning process, reward and punishment (or absence of reward), that is being proposed here. When spontaneous expression is "rewarded" (met adequately by maternal response), it (either the specific act or the fact of spontaneous expression itself) will tend to be repeated. The reverse—corresponding to failure in this early core development—entails repeated inadequate response to the child's spontaneous expression, such that these expressions become less likely to be emitted. Winnicott proposes that they are then replaced by actions of the child that are meant to accommodate to the world, at the expense of inner expression—the beginnings of a "false self." In this intrapsychic system, "ownership" of one's urges enhances the sense of "true self," giving it an additional fullness and force, widening the sense of "me" and "mine." The phenomenon that Modell (1984) discusses in terms of a patient's "having his own life," and the difficulties therein for some individuals, may well have some of its roots in such early true self–false self developments.

And a third, early, core development in the domain of self is that set of experiences having to do with the sense of well-being, of what will evolve into self-esteem when the sense of self, the "I," is more fully evolved (see Pine, 1982, for a fuller discussion of this). Kohut (1977) emphasizes in this the role of the parental inputs—the caretakers' smiling, rewarding responsiveness to the child's initiatives. The warmth and welcome of that response, by contrast, say, to a flat and depressed or a chiding and forbidding one, fills the child with a sense of goodness and worth. And, in terms of yet earlier phenomena, White (1963) and Broucek (1979) show how efficacy, competence, the ability to do, to make things happen, is an early bedrock of a sense of worth, of self-esteem.

And, last, core developmental phenomena in the domain addressed by a psychology of ego function: much of this is already implied in the discussions from the perspective of drive, object relations, and self. For the beginnings of delay and aim inhibition and other defense in respect to the drives is, from another perspective, a core development in the psychology of the ego—a basic task being the establishment of a reliable defense repertoire that can be called into play in the face of perceived threat. Another aspect of core development in relation to defense is the taking over, by the child, of the defense function—such that what was once *external* (that is, the caretaker as the primary protector against excess stimulation and pain) becomes *intrapsychic*, with the growing child more and more able to draw on his or her own (defense) resources. And core developments in ego function are also implied in the development of self-other differentiation, discussed in connection with the psychology of self experience, for such differentiation of self and other is one of the central achievements of reality testing, as Freud (1911) wrote, the distinction between inside and outside. And those developments that include the cognitive expansion of the "representational world," and the visual-motor achievements that underlie early efficacy and competence, and the expansion of affect and motility that help define the sense of self are all, from the current perspective, enlargements of the sphere of ego function—of adaptation, reality testing, and defense. The infant, early on, has brief moments of "alert inactivity" (Wolff, 1959) which are likely to be the times of its most advanced cognitive functioning, of its greatest attunement to the world "out there." If the infant and growing child, later, is not overwhelmed by anxiety and unsatisfied need (White, 1963), or, say, by panic over separateness (Mahler, 1968)—either of which can wash out and overrun the quiet times of alert inactivity—if the infant or child is *not* thus overwhelmed, the periods of alert inactivity (and later alert activity) can be seen to expand to fill most of the waking day, permitting the expansion of learning, of reality assessment, and, broadly, of the functioning of what we refer to as the ego.

To repeat my central argument: while developments in each of the four psychologies go on over the full life span, early developments in each nonetheless have a special status. That special status is what I have tried to convey here. It involves the whole construction of a differentiated intrapsychic life, of a conception of a self, a world, and a set of tools (action capabilities, understandings, expectations) that mediate between self and world; and along with this sense of an inner world, there is a capacity to "own" it, to express it, and to defend against aspects of it—or, of course, failures in any of these.

In conclusion, I pose the question whether development is seen as continuous or discontinuous, but I will not answer it in an either-or manner. I believe that such early developments as I have just described do have a special position in the life process, setting subsequent directions, opening up or limiting adaptive-expressive possibilities, defining core psychopathology; as such, there is a discontinuity in development—not in the sense that later development will not follow from this but in the sense that later development cannot have the same *impact*. Nonetheless, there is no single point when (say, after the first year, or two, or five, or whatever) we can say that these "early" developments reach a decisive end, nor is there ever a case in which they absolutely cannot be altered by subsequent developments.

LATER DEVELOPMENTS IN THE FOUR PSYCHOLOGIES

Earlier in this chapter I argued that the latency concept is one that is relevant only within the drive psychology; there is no latency in the development of ego, object relations, and self in this period. And latency is in fact the form of development within the drive psychology at this time, with shifts in drive-defense arrangements and with the progressive incorporation of residual issues of infantile sexuality into character style being the most prominent developments. The term *later* in this section refers to the entire life cycle, from childhood on, after the initial formative period discussed in the previous section.

There are two general features of the developmental process—one relatively widespread (at least within each culture) and one individual and particular—which serve to stimulate these later developments. The first has to do with some combination of biological maturation and cultural expectation that sets psychological tasks for each person at marker points along the chronological life path, each of these having the potential for requiring shifts in the individual's psychological organization—shifts that may affect phenomena addressed by any or all of the four psychologies. As early as 1950, Erikson had outlined one view of such development-linked "tasks" in his "eight stages of man." The other stimulus to such later changes is more individual; it comes from those inducements, elicitings, opportunities, or lost opportunities that individual history happens to bring into the life of one or another person. Rather than approaching this section by a discussion of each of the four psychologies taken one at a time, I shall approach it in terms of the general inducements to change that stem from the developmental process itself (in particular as addressed by various specific analytic writers) and in terms of the circumstances of individual histories. I shall start with the latter and with two relatively extreme examples.

We know that brainwashing or thought control can make for profound changes in the organization of the personality. Little has been written on this from the point of view of the drive psychology, and the defense organization in relation to drives, but much can be said of other sectors of the personality. A striking change is in the self organization, in particular in the nature of personal agency—of being the active agent in one's life. For the nature of that agency radically alters. The sense of being in charge of one's life may still be there; but the what and the how of the inner instructions by which one lives have profoundly changed. And this change in this aspect of the self organization is in turn reflective of profound changes in the object relations psychology—that is, in those objects that have been internalized as ideals and as models for conscience. Seen as a form of adaptation, the espousal of new beliefs can also be seen as reflective of major alterations within the psychology of the ego—as is, also, the marshaling of cognition and affect around the expression of those (new) beliefs.

Or, a second extreme example, the experience of the Holocaust by its most immediate victims—those in the death camps: while some have written about the maintenance of the sense of self through the continued operation of the prior (inner) life-style (Bettelheim, 1943) or about the continued humane concern for others among many in the camps, we also know of alterations in the internalized object relations and the drive organization (such as identification with the aggressor), of ego organization (such as denial), and of self organization (such as the centrality of humiliation) as significant ones among the potential outcomes.

I start with these two brief extreme examples only to highlight the point that later life experiences have the potential of inducing or requiring profound alterations in one or another aspect of an individual's functioning. But one does not have to go to such extreme situations to find instances of the same thing. We well know how, for some, the death of a long-term partner can lead to significant changes in the personal drive psychology—through the loss of the sexual partner to, say, a turning back upon masturbation and fantasy, or renewed searching for a partner with possible rearousal of all of the old sexual conflicts that had found a relatively settled (even if not "healthy") position with the formerly established partner. And, in most, the effect of such loss shows itself in mood—a point of contact between the self experience and the ego as the seat of affects. But more profound, from the point of view of ego function, are those alterations in cognitive function (memory and living in reality) and adaptation that one can see in the very old when a spouse is lost.

Or take the finding of a new mate, or the birth of a child, or the entry into new work: each of these provides new challenges and opportunities that may, in individual instances, foster and support the emergence of other aspects of the personality or, contrariwise, challenge established ways and lead to their deterioration. Just to select examples at random from an endless array of possibilities: the finding of a mate may incite pathological repetitions of old object relationships within that new relationship, or challenge the defense system (because of the demands of intimacy and sexuality) in ways that may lead to anxiety, new symptom formation, or even disorganization; or, contrariwise, it may lead to a heightening of self-esteem, a freeing of sexuality as conscience now gives permission, or a stimulus to higher levels of personal adaptation and achievement via new opportunities and new models. The birth of a child can also foster destructively renewed or reparatively revamped reenactments of old object relations or, through the intimacies of bodily care, a new sense of personal connectedness to others and of worth as one who can care for and be loved. Also, and on the other hand, parenthood brings new challenges—sometimes disruptive—to one's inner solution of oral, anal, or oedipal issues, as the child moves through those phases and restimulates old conflicts in the caretakers. And work, too, is not without such opportunities and challenges. The relative neutrality of relationships in the workplace can lead to a flowering of ego function not evident in more passionate relationships, or the competitiveness of the workplace can lead to the stimulation of oedipal, sadomasochistic, or other hostile or destructive fantasies that can produce failure or, on the other hand, adaptive character change. And particular work brings challenges by the contents of the work itself—the bodily intimacies faced by a physician (or, in different ways, by professional athletes), the psychological intimacies faced by analysts and therapists, the challenges to conscience faced by lawyers, the challenges of intimacy and sexuality faced by two police officers in a car alone together on patrol all day—not to mention the unconscious individualized meanings of particular work and of work itself to each person. All of these are but the tip of the iceberg of those countless challenges and opportunities of everyday life that can stimulate changes in the personal drive, ego, object relations, or self psychologies of any one person.

And a final illustration of such environmentally induced alterations is psychotherapy or psychoanalysis itself. For the very rationale of such treatment is based on the belief that later experiences can induce changes in significant aspects of functioning within the domains of each of the psychologies. Beyond the active work of the treatment, the relationship to the therapist/

analyst in itself, and the forms of activity required of the patient, themselves are mutative for aspects of the person—as discussed by James Strachey (1934) regarding superego alteration and Loewald (1960) regarding ego function and object relations (and see chapter 12).

So much by way of illustration of some of the inducements brought by individual history to later alterations in any or all of the personal psychologies of each individual. Let me turn now to such inducements—rather, requirements—built into the developmental process itself. I shall approach this by authors, rather than by each of the psychologies, to avoid the artificiality of too great a separation of the four, a separation which in any case cannot be seen clearly because of the interpenetration of the issues of all of the psychologies in character and personality by later ages. The first model for such a view of later developmental change is Freud's (1905) contribution itself, beginning with the charting of the early psychosexual stages, the latency period, and adolescence with its second coming of sexuality and, hence, its renewal of the residues of the first (infantile) sexuality. Changes in drive organization—in delay and control, in sublimation and aim inhibition, in "object removal" (Katan, 1951) and new object finding—are the defining features of this developmental line. And we can extend it to those alterations in sexual organization that are consequent upon mate finding in late adolescence and early adulthood, and to the changes of later life, such as menopause and, for both sexes (but often more disruptive for men, where it is heavily endowed with meanings for identity and self-esteem), the lessened intensity of the sexual urge.

As I described the range of developments within the several psychologies in the so-called latency period, Peter Blos (1962) has done this far more extensively for the adolescent period. His characterization of adolescence as the "second individuation phase" (1967) alludes to issues that I subsume under the psychologies of object relations and self experience, and his descriptions of the subphases of adolescence (1962) are organized centrally around changes in narcissism and object relations as well as forms of sexual expression. Most especially, his discussion of the reorganizations of late adolescence inevitably address core shifts in ego organization, goals and life tasks (built around attempted mastery of old trauma and internalized object relations), a relatively permanent sense of sexual identity and of preferred object choice, and, of course, preferred forms and tolerable limits of sexual expression. Clearly, in adolescence, as in childhood and earlier, continued major changes in functioning take place—expressible in the languages of the four psychologies.

Nathan Segel (1981) describes lifespan changes relevant to "narcissism and adaptation to indignity." In spite of the focus set by that title, the developments he includes spread far beyond narcissism, though he views them from that vantage point. He writes:

[This] brings me to the very last part of this paper, where I can only briefly refer to aspects of a subject that might warrant a paper by itself, i.e., our increasing awareness of the role of narcissism throughout all the developmental phases, not as an exclusive manifestation of the Psychology of the Self, but as a result of our broadened understanding of the necessity to incorporate the role of self needs among those of object needs. For the adult as well as the child, life brings with it phase specific needs for all of us to make adaptations to the indignity that life can bestow. It is how we adjust to these indignities, and even whether we can abstract from them further adaptive structures and strength that will determine at each stage the ultimate status of our self-esteem regulation as well as our relations with objects. Mahler (1975) and Settlage (1977) have beautifully delineated developmental conflicts going back to the "practicing period" of separation-individuation and the traumatic vulnerability of the child's narcissism at the point when his delusion of omnipotence is at its peak and also most vulnerable to the dangers of deflation from a new and disturbing reality which will climax in the "rapprochement crisis." Similarly, it seems to me, the child who is lifted up high by an adoring, empathic father and then unsuccessfully attempts to lift this parent in turn, is face to face with the need to cope with a narcissistically traumatic event, regardless of how empathic the idealizing parental image is. There is an intrapsychic conflict here related to ambivalence and deflation and not just a trauma due to empathic failure. The child who wishes to replace the envied parent of the opposite sex, or the adolescent who wishes to impose his rule on the world at a time when he still doesn't even have a vote, all face the task of adaptation to such indignities. In later life the need to cope with various aspects of waning physical functions and strength, or accepting a younger rival as one's boss, and ultimately even the possibility of coping with loss of control of bodily functions, are just a tiny sampling of life's indignities which almost all of us will encounter at some stage. For all of us engaged in clinical work, it may be especially relevant to be reminded that one of the greatest indignities is regularly endured by our patients, no matter how gently we cushion the blow, or how much we strain our empathic resources. I am referring here to the indignity of being an adult in therapy, while simultaneously allowing the emergence, in the transference, of infantile aspects of ourselves that the adult part of ourselves experiences as so humiliating and demeaning, *and further*, having to share it with another adult. For this reason, if for none better, it behooves us all to understand as much as possible about normal narcissism and its vicissitudes throughout life in our relationship to objects as well as to ourselves. (pp. 473–474)

Elsewhere (Pine, in press), I have taken a similar life-span perspective on the place of object loss in normal development. There, too, while I do not focus on the issue specifically from the viewpoint of the four psychologies, it is clear that the forms of object loss are stage-related (and therefore built in and inevitable) and act as inducements to change in the full array of phenomena addressed by the several psychologies. The forms of object loss that I discuss in that paper include: the loss of the illusion of oneness in infancy, the loss (through intrapsychic changes) of the parents-of-childhood in adolescence, and in adulthood, the losses of omnipotentiality (the sense that all life possibilities are open to oneself) and, later, of optimal bodily function or appearance (both losses of the self as object), and the losses of one's children (through growth) and of one's love objects (through death), both losses of the other as object. Among these are specific inducements to changes in aspects of internalized object relations (centrally) but also of self experience, drive organization, and ego function.

And let me come last to the one who came first in terms of analytic views of life span development: namely, Erikson (1950). He lists eight of what he refers to as "ego qualities—criteria by which the individual demonstrates that his ego, at a given stage, is strong enough to integrate the timetable of the organism with the structure of social institutions" (p. 218). The well-known list of pairings includes: trust versus basic mistrust (in the "oral-sensory" period), autonomy versus shame and doubt (in the "anal-muscular" period), initiative versus guilt (in the "locomotor-genital" period), industry versus inferiority (in the latency period), identity versus role diffusion (in puberty and adolescence), intimacy versus isolation (in young adulthood), and generativity versus stagnation and then integrity versus despair (in later stages of adulthood). I list them here because, although Erikson offers them as "ego qualities" indicating the capacity to "integrate" organismic and social demands, what they reflect and integrate can readily be seen to be reflective of phenomena in each of the several psychologies. Thus—as examples and with no attempt at completeness—the trust versus mistrust issue at minimum is built on early object attachment and expectation of reliable tension relief and drive gratification; the identity versus role diffusion issue revolves not only around resolution of sexual identity and object relations as worked through in adolescence, but additionally (in terms of the emphases in some of the current literature) around individuation, self-organization, and self-esteem; and generativity versus stagnation is built around continued success in sublimation and flexibility of defense organization and on ego organization and satisfaction within the sphere of object relations more broadly. We could proceed in like manner for each of the paired ego qualities.

It is not only possible developmentally, but also useful clinically, to view the developmental process as one wherein life (development and circumstance) presents the individual with a series of successive challenges ("tasks") which the individual meets in part in new ways and in part by trying to absorb them into old ways of functioning. Anna Freud (1936) described this graphically in her discussion of two alternative forms of pathological moves from latency into adolescence: in one the defense structure crumbles and in the other it remains immovable, the person retaining a latency-like organization throughout life, making no room for the newfound sexuality of adolescence. The "tasks" of development are numerous, including self-differentiation, object attachment, and defense development early on; the move into peer relations, learning, and the displacements and sublimations that are tied to those in the latency period; the inclusion of sexuality in the personality and the definitive shift to nonfamilial objects for sexual and affective life in adolescence; adult attachment, childrearing, and work in early and mid-adulthood; and loss and decline in old age. Each individual meets each of these developmental challenges in part by the effort to *assimilate* them—that is, to bring to bear one's familiar mode of functioning in the drive, ego, object relations, and self spheres and make the new situation into a continuation of the old. In fact, just as the past is seen reenacted in the transference, so too is it reenacted upon new life events in the effort to absorb them into old and familiar ways. On the other hand, there is always some *accommodation*—some shift of the internal organization in the direction required for adaptation to the new challenges. These stimulate change in the organization of the personal psychologies at significant steps along the developmental pathway, and this is part of what I refer to as life-span development in each of the four domains.

In summary, my main point in this chapter has been twofold: the overarching one is that a four psychologies view of the developmental process throughout the life cycle is both plausible and useful, and is the underpinning for the argument for the clinical utility of that same four psychologies view advanced in the previous chapter; and the second point is that, within the life-span developmental view of the four psychologies, early developments in each of the four have a special place in producing (in various terms, to capture the spirit of it) the creation of an intrapsychic life, the structuralization of the personality, and an individual that enters as a causal agent in his or her own life stream because of the establishment of preference, specific repetitions, mechanisms, and structural limitations.

Developments within each of the psychologies include also the development of distinctive motivations characteristic of each. I have reserved that discussion for the next chapter.

CHAPTER 5

The Development of Motivation

THROUGHOUT HIS WRITINGS, Freud focused on the central task of defining the core motivations that govern human intrapsychic life and, through that, human behavior. He tended to think in dualisms and at various times drew on sexual drives, ego instincts, self- and species-preservation, narcissism, and life (eros) and death (thanatos) instincts—the last including the repetition compulsion "beyond the pleasure principle" (Freud, 1920a). The final form of the motivational dualism as most analysts have worked with it for the better part of this century is the dualism of sexuality and aggression, the former an "instinctual drive" and the latter of somewhat less clear conceptual status.

In this chapter I propose a wider array of motives that govern human behavior—motives within each of the four psychologies. I see this array as clinically relevant, and my interest in them grew from what I see in the clinical situation. But I shall pursue their formation in the development of the individual, attempting to show both their biological origins and ultimately their psychoanalytic and clinical relevance as motives. My approach will be developmental throughout, asking, how are motives born in the course of development? In answering this question, I shall propose that all human motives have a developmental history. Whatever the nature of their initial biological base, the final forms of motivation are the result of complex shaping processes that take time to occur. Thus the relevant question is how motivational status is achieved *over time*. My take-off point and my focus remain the clinical situation, and it is the developmentally evolved, not the biologically programmed, forms of motivation that have significance there.

A particular theoretical point would flow from a successful argument that quite different motives govern intrapsychic life in the domains of each of the psychologies. For if it can be shown that phenomena of each of the four psychologies achieve motivational status, then each can be viewed somewhat more as a relatively independent actor on the intrapsychic stage. This would tend to differentiate the four psychologies further, pushing them beyond the point of being simply points of view or reducible to one or another.

When behavior seems to be sustained and organized around specific aims of the individual, we think of it as motivated. Or, in reverse, "motivation equals all variables which arouse, sustain, and direct behavior" (Madsen, 1959, p. 44). In this sense, there are motives specific to the domains of each of the four psychologies, and one cannot render a comprehensive account of mental life without taking each of them into account. In describing how behavior is thus "aroused, sustained, and directed," I shall postulate a variety of forms of motivation—self-initiating ("proactive"), reactive, and homeostatic—each having differing subforms as well. As suggested above, such differences in the nature of motivation in the domains of each of the psychologies help underwrite the claim that they are indeed different psychologies; a person may be under the sway of quite different kinds of motives at different times.

In response to an argument along these lines, when Robert White (1959, 1963) introduced his concept of "effectance" motivation, Rapaport (1960a) offered a distinction between motives and other causes of behavior. Motives, he argued, are "*appetitive* internal forces" (p. 865)—peremptory, cyclic, selective, and displaceable—a description particularly apt for instinctual drives. I shall work with the broader rather than the narrower definition of motives ("all variables which arouse, sustain, and direct behavior" rather than "appetitive internal forces"). There is potential gain for clinical work in recognizing the quite different forms of motivation in the domains of the several psychologies.

MOTIVATION IN THE FOUR PSYCHOLOGIES

Object Relations Psychology

I should like to approach the issue of motivation within the object relations psychology in two ways: first via general background considerations and second via the clinical situation.

Classical analytic drive theory has essentially two views with regard to the early relationship to the object. First, the object is seen as the means through which gratification is achieved—that is, as the end point of the drive's action. And second, the object is seen as coming to be important because a particular object, the primary caretaker, is associated with drive gratification —that is, it is a conditioned stimulus.

Others since have argued for the primacy of attachment to the object— that is, primacy in that it is prewired, there from the start, and not dependent on association with drive gratification. In Fairbairn's (1941) aphorism, drives are object seeking, not pleasure seeking. For Bowlby (1969), who marshals considerable argument and evidence to sustain his point, object attachment is primary but can be best understood in terms of "the environment of evolutionary adaptedness" (pp. 58–64)—the time when survival for early man, living in the wild and near the danger of animal attack, would be enhanced by attachment to the group which lessened the dangers of wandering off into darkness and danger from other animals. Thus, he argues, attachment had (and has) survival value; given that fact, and given the widespread nature of fear of the dark, of separation anxiety, and of stranger anxiety, it makes sense to think of object attachment as a primary, built-in feature of human functioning. And Stern's (1985) recent review of the infant literature, and his own work, makes clear that object attachment, of remarkable subtlety and substantiality, is present so early as to render forced and artificial any attempt to explain this as being *derived* from drive gratification in some secondary way.

From one point of view, all of these arguments just bear on the chicken-

and-egg problem: which comes first, drive gratification or object attachment? And in that form the argument is not productive. Even if we could ascertain whether one or another came first, it is clear that from very early on they are each already present and are en route on a complex developmental path, intertwined with one another, such that nothing significant about human functioning can be described without reference to both. And from my point of view, developed earlier, it is easy to conceive of and to identify some moments that are relatively more organized in terms of drive gratification, and others that are relatively more organized in terms of object interconnection, even from very early on. Since these organizations are momentary (and changing), there is time and place for each of them—and more.

But from a second point of view, the question of a biologically built-in basic attachment to the object (Bowlby, 1969) bears on a central phenomenon of object relations theories in psychoanalysis, and links the biology of the organism to the psychology of the object tie. Specifically, I have in mind the phenomenon of the (ordinarily present) continued attachment to the primary objects of infancy no matter how "bad" these objects are experienced as being. The core attachment to them does not ordinarily decondition and disappear, but remains—a measure, perhaps, of the moments of gratification (positive reinforcement) that must have inevitably been present if the infant were to survive but also, perhaps, of the built-in nature of the earliest ties. This would be somewhat along the lines of an imprinting response (Lorenz, 1965, 1970) but, of course, subject to vastly greater developmental variation in an organism as complex as the human being.

The issue of motivation in relation to object relations as we see it in the clinical situation is at quite a different level from such questions of early pre-wiring or conditioning, and is best understood in terms of the *tendency to repeat* (Freud, 1920a). When Robert Waelder (1936) advanced his concept of multiple function, he suggested that all behaviors have functions in relation to drive gratification, adaptation, conscience, and repetition. The first three were clear even then, and are continually confirmed in the clinical situation; they are not relevant for my present discussion, and I shall not discuss them further here. But what of repetition? It is not so immediately evident that all behaviors have functions in relation to repetition. For Freud, repetition was understood in two quite different ways. One of these, a biophysical speculation, had to do with energic tendencies for return to quiescence—a psychic entropy—a view that led to his formulation of the death instinct. But such a speculation is at a level radically different from that of the functions of behavior in relation to drive gratification, adaptation, and conscience—each of which can readily be seen in the clinical situation. Freud's other use of repetition was based on his observation that trauma, defined as levels of stimulus input too great to be mastered at the time of input, are repeated actively in (automatic) efforts after mastery. A readily available illustration is of someone telling and retelling the story of an operation or accident until internal quiescence, mastery, is achieved. This view of repetition, while it seems to be applicable not universally to all behaviors but only to those of a traumatic nature, nonetheless points to a place for an omnipresent tendency to repeat as well as to the motivational force in the object relations domain.

I have in mind the proposal, discussed earlier (Pine, 1985), that there is a universal tendency actively to repeat old internalized object relations. I am referring to object relations *as experienced* (not veridical) and as recorded in memory—in the representational world (Sandler and Rosenblatt, 1962) of images, actions, and expectations. I am not blind to the fact that the repetitions of old object relations often have an automatic, unconsciously propelled character. We see the patient's behavior, for example, and only much later in an analysis discover the ways in which it is a repetition. But it is an *active* repetition in the sense that it is *motivated*, transformative of or connecting to the old object relationship (see Loewald's [1971b] discussion of repetition).

What are the forces behind those tendencies to repeat—that is, where does the motivational force come from? Pleasure and trauma, two familiar sources. Thus, there is a tendency to repeat old internalized object relations because they have a traumatic aspect—not usually all-at-once overwhelming trauma ("shock" trauma, in Kris's [1956a] sense), but the slowly accruing, disturbing, irritating trauma (Kris's "strain" trauma) that accumulates over a lifetime of at least partially distressing familial relationships for the child. From this standpoint, old internalized (experienced) object relations are seen to be repeated in efforts at mastery, the effort to turn the old passive experience into an active one—whether done to others or "actively" (though unconsciously) done to oneself. I have found interpretations along these lines to have powerful impact upon patients. And the pleasure aspect? Old internalized object relations are also repeated in efforts at pleasure—

pleasure because they represent the attachment to the parents of childhood, and repetition (unconsciously) keeps those relationships alive. Enactment makes them real in the here and now. But these "pleasures," seen in the clinical situation, often are virtually identical with the strain-traumatic attachment to old objects. That is, they are the pleasures of attachment to the only parents one has had, and in this sense pleasurable whether "objectively" built around apparently good or apparently bad experiences. That particular goodness or badness is not for the outsider to judge; it is the experiencing subject's mode of connection. And here we can see that repetition in efforts at mastery of the strain trauma or in efforts after pleasure frequently merge with one another. For the pleasure of attachment may involve the same behaviors that are irritant-level traumas or worse, and which are repeated to rid oneself of the passive position. In my clinical experience, it seems to me that this blending is generally the case with regard to the significant phenomena of a psychoanalysis.

So I propose repetition in the effort at mastery of the strain trauma in old object relationships as a primary and the most distinctive motive force in the domain of the object relations psychology at the clinically relevant level, and suggest that it is omnipresent, powerful, and conceptually sufficient to do the job (explaining the proactive, behavior-organizing, directive features of the object relations psychology) that I am calling upon it to do.

Clearly there is also place for the motive force of more purely pleasurable attachment seeking. This motive is often, but not always, a reflection of drive-derived wishes in relation to the object as well. This area has been most fully explored by Joseph and Anne-Marie Sandler (1978; Sandler, 1976, 1981). They wrote:

> The child who has a wish to cling to the mother has, as part of this wish, a mental representation of himself clinging to the mother. But he also has, in the content of his wish, a representation of the mother or her substitute responding to his clinging in a particular way, possibly by bending down and embracing him. This formulation is rather different from the idea of a wish consisting of a wishful aim being directed towards an object. The idea of an aim which seeks gratification has to be supplemented by the idea of a *wished-for interaction*, with the wished-for or imagined response of the object being as much a part of the wishful fantasy as the activity of the subject in that wish or fantasy. (p. 288)

Thus, here, the argument is advanced for pleasure-based efforts toward repetition of old object relations. But the argument does not rest at this point. Thus, Sandler (1981) writes:

Just as the tension produced by drive stimuli may evoke wishes, so can other stimuli (e.g., external stimuli) call forth the wish. If, for some reason, there is a lessening of our background feeling of safety, appropriate wishes to do something which would restore that feeling of security are evoked. If self-esteem is threatened, compensatory narcissistic wishful fantasies may result. . . . The pain of loss will evoke wishes to restore the relation to the lost object in some way. Anxiety in its various forms (I include feelings of shame and guilt) is a most potent stimulus to wishful activity, the aim of the wish being to restore feelings of well-being. . . . I want to stress that wishes to establish and reestablish certain types of relationship with others need not be motivated by sexual or aggressive drives alone, but may primarily represent attempts to restore or maintain feelings of well-being and security. (p. 188)

In this argument, as advanced, it can be seen that repetition of earlier object relationships can serve motivational aims (in my terms, as I shall develop them later) related to the domain of the ego psychology (stilling anxiety), of the psychology of self experience (restoring a state of narcissistic well-being), or of the drive psychology (gratification of libidinal wishes). Though, for the sake of explication, I describe the psychologies separately, in human functioning they are, of course, integrated (and see chapter 6 on this). And I repeat what I said earlier, that a primary and the most distinctive motive force specific to the domain of the object relations psychology is repetition in the effort at mastery of the strain trauma in those experienced object relationships themselves.

The Psychology of Self Experience

In the infant and young child there is gradually built up a sense of a self, a familiar self of particular boundaries, continuity, valuation, and overall subjective state. If something *feels* wrong in this primary self feeling, attention turns to that, with efforts of some sort to right that ill feeling. This is essentially a view of motivation as homeostatic and built around constant fine tuning based upon subjective state. Let me clarify and expand upon it.

We assume that there is a development early on, at some pace, of self-awareness—of recognition of "I" and its familiar states. The timetable of this development has been written about by numerous authors (Spitz, 1957; Mahler, 1972; Pine, 1982; Stern, 1985), but the actual timetable is not relevant to my argument. What *is* central, however, is that at some point there comes into being for every individual a sense of self-recognition built around familiar and ongoing subjective states and that certain forms of interruption or threatened interruption of those states trigger attempts to maintain the (psychological) steady state—to maintain homeostasis. The forms and tolerance levels of the particular subjective state will naturally vary over time, but the homeostatic tendencies nonetheless remain present.

Homeostatic mechanisms at the subjective psychological level, just as at the physiological level, are an evolutionary necessity. The infant's cry, when in subjective discomfort, is a built-in warning sign notifying the caretaker that something is out of balance. This is a prewired adaptive mechanism; it alerts the caretaker to act to help to reintroduce homeostasis—most typically, in the newborn, to satisfy hunger. The mechanism remains the same later on, though the subjective state will alter from biological hunger to quite different forms of *self* experience; earlier I proposed that these include boundaries, continuity and wholeness, authenticity, agency, and self-valuation (esteem). And the cry is replaced by more subtle inner mechanisms, such as coercion of the mother, or delusion (to deny differentiated boundaries), or accentuating character differences (Pine, 1979b) to preserve those boundaries, or in another domain, mechanisms such as grandiosity or abasement to affect self-valuation. My point is that, early on, subjective discomfort is a momentary state, short-lived, and the homeostatic need is terminated as soon as relief comes. But, later on, when there is ongoing awareness of a preferred subjective self-state, a kind of self-constancy, then the homeostatic need—that is, the automatic effort to right imbalances in that subjective state—also becomes ongoing, becomes a lasting pressure to act in certain ways to maintain the preferred self-state (see Sandler, 1960).

What I am proposing here has its parallel in what I shall propose below regarding the aggressive drive, following John McDevitt (1980, 1983); there I shall argue that the brief aggressive reaction acquires ongoingness, lasting quality, with the development of object constancy—when the offending other can be held in mind. For the regulation of self-state (parallel to aggression), an ongoing motive quality (rather than the simple reflex-like reaction, say, to hunger) comes into being when a sense of "I," or self-constancy (parallel to object constancy) is held in mind. At that point, continuously acting motives, triggered by homeostatic imbalances, begin to develop to regulate that self-state.

The best approximation I can give to the significant parameters of the familiar self-state, based on contributions available in the psychoanalytic literature, includes whatever degree of boundary differentiation (varying from sharply etched to nonexistent, with all intermediate points possible as well) is subjectively comfortable for that individual, the nature and degree of worth (esteem) in one's own subjective sense and in relations (real and imagined) with others, the sense of authenticity and agency (a "true self" living one's own life), and the sense of wholeness/fragmentation or continuity/discontinuity—overall, of integration—of the experienced self. There is nothing sacred about this way of describing the central lines of the subjective self; these reflect abstractions from the current literature. But it is at the core of this proposal that there be *some* central parameters to the ongoing subjective sense of self, probably varying from person to person, and that alterations in this familiar and comfortable state lead to active attempts to reestablish the familiar state. Call these narcissistic adaptations or defenses, if you will. The name is less important than the phenomenon. But I should add that the particular familiar and comfortable subjective steady state favored by an individual need not be "healthy" in the clinician's eye. For one person, shadowy self-other boundaries are comfortable and awareness of differentiation is a threat; for another, an abased self-image; and so forth.

Throughout the discussion in this chapter I have been assuming that core human motives need not be present from birth, but are formed in varying ways in the course of development. (Homeostatic tendencies are, of course, part of all living systems and in that sense universal; but here I am attempting to describe the development of an active motive.) Significant psychological phenomena can come into being at many stages of the life cycle and can then achieve a status as independent factors ("causes") in the determination of behavior. So, too, I propose here. Whenever, and on the basis of whatever contents, a familiar and comfortable subjective sense of self is attained, when there is an "I" and it has specific form, interruptions to that state will lead generally to vigorous attempts to right it. These attempts have motivational force and are, I propose, the significant motives with regard to self experience, the domain of the subjective sense of self. And the coming into being of this motive gives force to the psychology of self experience, making it a significant additional factor in psychic life.

The motivation to maintain the comfortable subjective steady state will not be equally apparent in every person. Things that work smoothly are scarcely noticed. Thus, effectively operating intrapsychic defenses and smoothly working reality testing are scarcely noticed; there is no "effort," for example, to "test reality"; it just happens. For some, the ongoing subjective state of self, as I have defined its parameters here, is relatively stable and needs little more than fine tuning. But for those who have not established a basic awareness of differentiation from others, ultimately rooted in realistic perception, and for those who have not comfortably settled their use of others as selfobjects (Kohut, 1977) but for whom this remains a stress-filled aspect of functioning, and for those whose esteem is constantly dependent upon inputs from the outside—for all of those, the subjective state of self will be at constant risk in all interpersonal interactions (as well as in alone states), and the need to right the subjective state of self (whether through grandiosity, omnipotence, denial, clinging, manipulation, or whatever) will be a constant and central task.

Ego Psychology

Earlier I defined the domain of the ego psychology as involving those behaviors having to do with reality testing, adaptation, and defense. These certainly start from a biological base. We can no longer fail to give recognition to the fact that the human infant is governed by a tendency toward stimulus seeking as well as tension reduction (see White, 1963; Lichtenberg, 1983). The recent flood of experimental infant research (Stone, Smith and Murphy, 1973; Osofsky, 1979; Stern, 1985) makes clear that, virtually from the start of postuterine life, the infant's perceptual apparatus is attuned to the outside with consequences for memory, learning, and cognition more broadly. That is, what we conceive of as reality attunement and adaptation is built upon prewired aspects of the infant organism. So, too, is defense (defined broadly as tension regulation). Joseph Lichtenberg (1983) summarizes it thus: "What is suggested by the research [on the neonate] is that rather than a stimulus barrier and simple [tension] reduction mechanism, the newborn is innately equipped to *regulate* stimuli and tension within optimal threshold limits" (p. 6). "Competence" (White, 1963), the capacity to make things happen, is an outgrowth of such prewired tendencies and is a bedrock of self-esteem. The relevant point for motivation theory is that reality testing and adaptation have a self-propelled quality. Though conflict, search for drive gratification, and ties to the object affect them profoundly, they start from a built-in base. Put otherwise, the built-in tendency toward exploration and learning leads to a *base* for, for instance, reality testing (through perception and memory) and self-esteem (through the ability to produce an effect, to make things happen), so that when these develop out of conflict or object relational processes (such as mirroring or identification), there is already a core present; they do not have to start from scratch. All through development, we see later editions of this built-in tendency to exercise newfound functions ("function-lust" in Ives Hendrick's [1942] term): the toddler's constant locomotion and soon thereafter the constant use of verbalization to name things or to ask questions, the tendency to exercise skills, whether in athletics, painting, writing, dancing, or what have you. Though we well know that psychoanalytic listening will reveal a conflict- and drive-related component of such exercise of skills, this need not lead us to a reductionistic view. There is every reason to assume that the complex neurological apparatus given to us by evolution is preset to function at least in some important ways in relation to the environment in which it evolved.

Once again, the biological base, here the built-in ego apparatuses (Hartmann, 1939) that ensure responsiveness to stimuli and a self-propelled functioning "ego" (that is, tendencies toward reality testing, adaptation, and defense), is relevant to but quite different from the conception of motivation that we bring to bear on the clinical situation. For the early work of reality testing, adaptation, and of course defense involves just that: *work*. Because the infant is responsive to stimuli from within and without, there is distress involved again and again as efforts are made to meet and regularize (make predictable) that world of stimulation. Once some order, some predictability, some way of anticipating and mastering stimulation, is achieved, we can expect that that achievement will not readily be given up—again making for a tendency toward holding on to *sameness*.

Thus, I would propose that the clinically relevant motive as evolved in the domain of the ego psychology is the tendency of the ego to maintain its own organization in the effort to avoid negative affect; or, to state it with less reification of "the ego," the tendency of the person to continue to function in his or her familiar, and generally quite automatic, ways in order to avoid psychic pain. This has kinship to the homeostatic principle advanced earlier for the psychology of self experience—the tendency to retain a steady subjective state of self—but, in the present case, we are speaking of an area where the subjective phenomenological referents are less clear. Instead, the concept is based on inferences regarding personality organization (see Greenwald, 1980).

Though hard to pinpoint, it seems that we have not been able to do without such a concept (of maintenance of achieved organization); it appears frequently. The concept of resistance in clinical psychoanalysis gives recognition to the powerful forces opposing change. The concept of character gives recognition to the tendency, in each of us in our own way, to receive stimulation from within or without and make it into a kind of familiar sameness, to handle it in "characteristic" ways. A general fear of the strange would also bear on this general tendency to maintain sameness.

Waelder (1936) deals with this as well in his paper on multiple function:

> The ego appears to be solicited by concrete problems from four directions: from the outside world, from the compulsion to repeat, from the id, and from the superego. However, the role of the ego is not limited to this passivity alone. . . . Rather, it develops toward the outer world, as well as toward the other agencies in man himself, its own peculiar activity. This activity may be characterized as *striving to hold its own*, and beyond this to assimilate in organic growth the outer world as well as the other agencies within the ego. . . .
>
> The function of the ego is therefore not limited to finding attempted solutions for problems which are placed before it by the outer world, by the compulsion to repeat, by the id, by the superego, but in addition it assigns to itself definite problems, such as *overcoming the other agencies or joining them to its organization by active assimilation*. (pp. 47–48) [Emphasis added.]

Anna Freud (1936) struggled with the same issue. In discussing the basis for defense against instinct (including "superego anxiety" and "objective anxiety"), she adds "instinctual anxiety (dread of the strength of the instincts)" (p. 63). She goes on as follows:

The human ego by its very nature is never a promising soil for the unhampered gratification of instinct. I mean by this that the ego is friendly to the instincts, only so long as it is itself but little differentiated from the id. When it has evolved from the primary to the secondary process, from the pleasure-principle to the reality-principle, it has become, as I have already shown, alien territory to the instincts. Its mistrust of their demands is always present but, under normal conditions, hardly noticeable. It is lost sight of in the much more tumultuous warfare waged within its domain by the super-ego and the outside world against the impulses of the id. But, if the ego feels itself abandoned by these protective higher powers or if the demands of the instinctual impulses become excessive, its mute hostility to instinct is intensified to the point of anxiety. "What it is that the ego fears either from an external or from a libidinal danger cannot be specified; we know that it is in the nature of an overthrow or of extinction, but it is not determined by analysis" (Freud, 1923, p. 57). Robert Waelder describes it as "the danger that the ego's whole organization may be destroyed or submerged." (1936, p. 48)

In a recent fiftieth anniversary discussion of Freud's "Analysis Terminable and Interminable" (1937), Cooper (1987b) advances a similar argument:

Many contemporary analysts would add [to Freud's statement that the ego treats recovery itself as a new danger] that the prospect of change is viewed as a danger by the neurotic ego not only because it threatens the awakening of forbidden impulses, but because any change of ego function or attitude threatens the sense of safety and coherence represented by the habitual and familiar. As Freud himself points out (1937, p. 238), "the adult's ego . . . finds itself compelled to seek out those situations in reality which can serve as an approximate substitute for the original danger, *so as to be able to justify, in relation to them, its maintaining its habitual modes of reaction.*" [Emphasis added by Cooper.] One might interpret this as indicating that the ego is more concerned with its own coherence and consistency than with the original danger. (p. 135)

While this tendency of the ego to maintain its own organization can be viewed as nothing but the expression of, say, defense against drives, one's stand on this issue is probably, ultimately, a matter of theoretical preference. Certainly it can be seen as propelled by anxieties related to loss of the object, of the object's love, bodily damage, or superego condemnation—the traditional core anxieties. But it is also clear that the several authors quoted are trying to reach beyond that. It may be a characteristic of organized states (as of organizations altogether) that they tend toward a certain inertia (that is, a steady state unless actively forced to change). I propose that, once a particular and characteristic form of organization, a way of modulating stimuli, is achieved by each individual, the maintenance of that organization (within limits, and slowly evolving) itself becomes an independent force in personal functioning. The personal view of reality, and the mode of adaptation and defense, tend to be self-sustaining, to be maintained by the individual—sometimes, it seems, at all costs. It is perhaps most clear in the fragile individual's desperate clinging to his or her preferred internal order. This tendency to maintain the achieved mode of organization is central to the clinically relevant level of motivation in the domain of the ego psychology.

Drive Psychology

Though the sexual drives could be seen as the prototype of those variables (motives) that "arouse, sustain, and direct behavior," the motivational picture in this domain is nonetheless neither clear nor simple. Human beings can be single-minded in their pursuit of sexual gratification, organizing all perception, thought, and action in its direction, once arousal has been initiated; and the "driving" aspect here, that is the motivational feature, appears to be relatively clear cut phenomenologically. A sense of urgency, of peremptoriness, plus the capacity for sensual pleasure (see Klein, 1976), forms the biological substrate for the drive aspect of sexuality. And this sense of urgency can be attached to oral, anal, and genital erotogenic zones, as well as to the skin surface altogether. But clearly this biological substrate is, once again, just the beginning of a clinically relevant and developmentally shaped picture of motivation with regard to sexuality.

In the first place, it is in the nature of the human psyche that such sensations receive mental representation—they are recorded in perception, thought, and memory and attached to experiences. Specific forms of sensual stimulation received by the infant via the caretaker or from his or her own body are recorded in memory and begin to shape what we refer to as wishes in Freud's sense (1900), that is, the connection of an arousal to a memory of a previous satisfaction. As these, gradually and inevitably, become less veridical, taking bits and pieces from multiple experiences, and are altered by imagination and wishful distortion, they can better be described as fantasies than memories—that is, the wrapping of an arousal in a complex set of thoughts that can be experienced as a wish or a desire and that represent the mental conditions for satisfaction (see Sandler and Sandler, 1978). Sexual drives include the biological givens of bodily sensation but include also a record of personal history embodied in cognitions (wishes, fantasies, goals) that guide the form of arousal and satisfaction; they are not simply urges automatically played out.

And in the second place, what appears to be, and even includes, primary sexual motivation serves diverse aims (Klein, 1976, chap. 3). This outcome is inevitable, once we recognize the link of urge to cognition. Thus (and drawing on Klein's basic ideas but phrased in terms of the several psychologies) the urgency of the search for sensual experience of one kind or another may reflect its use for the "ego's" defensive purposes (say, to ward off another urge or to defend against negative affect), or in the repetition of an aspect of an old object relationship in the service of mastery, or to stabilize a disintegrating or abased sense of self.

In its least overdetermined form, sexual drive is relatively proactive (self-initiating), as opposed to reactive—though it can of course be triggered by external stimuli (see Holt, 1976). Its cyclic and peremptory quality stems from its bodily base. And the especially intense quality of sensual pleasure ensures the wish for its repetition (though, of course, conflict and defense alter this significantly). Behavior becomes organized in relation to it until satisfaction or some other route to quiescence is achieved, and this represents its "force" or motivational feature. However, while cyclicity, peremptoriness, and potential pleasure may account for the primary motivational aspect of sexuality, the omnipresence of the search for sensual pleasure requires a recognition of the functions it serves within the spheres of ego, object relations, and self experience as well. This is common knowledge within the interpretive work of clinical psychoanalysis; sensual pleasure serves many functions besides the attainment of pleasure in itself.

Parallel considerations—a built-in biological base, the role of learning and an expansion of functions to the areas of ego mastery, object relatedness, and self experience—are relevant regarding aggressive drive as well.

An aggressive urge can also serve as an organizer of behavior, giving it direction until some goal (release or satisfaction or defense against it) is attained. The proactive (as opposed to reactive) forms of aggression are not as clear, though it has been suggested that they are present in constructive "aggression" (mastery, exploration) (Parens, 1979; McDevitt, 1983). Its bodily source and its cyclic nature are also not compellingly clear, and it is fair to say that agreement regarding aggressive drive is not as widespread in the literature as is agreement in relation to sexual urges. But when we look to our animal forebears, we see that aggressive attack is linked to food getting, mate getting, and cub protection, as well as to territoriality more broadly. In these instances, there is a proactive aspect to aggression, as it is linked to other activities—and in humans this has been linked to oral biting, to anal sadism, and to phallic intrusiveness as well as to mastery. Such early experiences of aggressivity, tied as they are to pleasure as well, and embedded in early object relationships, are, through those ties, ensured a lasting place within individual wish and fantasy systems. Additionally, they provide a groundwork for other forms of aggression to be built upon.

These other forms are equally significant for us. They are largely reactive and they come in response to physical restraint even early on, and later to other interferences with directed activity (taking a toy away, getting in one's way); and also they come in response to frustrations of all kinds, including the denial of satisfaction and hurts to the self—"narcissistic injury." Though these forms of aggression are *reactive*, they are no less omnipresent than the proactive (cyclic) sexual drives or the aggressive actions that are inherently tied to biting, defecating, or other bodily functioning; this is so because there is no way in human life to avoid such interferences, frustrations, and hurts, and so reactive aggression is nonetheless universal. For the forms of aggression I am now addressing, the proactive, self-producing, cyclic aspects seem less central while the interferences, frustrations, and hurts of everyday life seem to provide their main source.

But how does such reactive aggression become a drive? How does it achieve ongoing motivational status? How does it become more than momentary? Here we have to recognize one of the mixed blessings of the human psychic apparatus: in the colloquial, the capacity to hold a grudge.

Let me take a detour by way of explanation. McDevitt (1980, 1983) reports an important set of infant observations. He found that early aggressive outbursts were reactive and short-lived. When the source of interference or frustration terminated, the aggressive response terminated. But after eighteen months or so, this was no longer as fully the case. Aggressive and angry reactions were sustained over time. He links this to the development of object constancy occurring at around the same time. That is, the toddler could presumably hold onto the idea of the frustrator after the specific frustration terminated. The aggressive response, now filtered through a more advanced cognitive system capable of differentiated perception of the source of injury and of memory of that source, could be retained over time. But here, then, we have the construction of an aggressive drive—beginning reactively, but held over time. It, too, like sexuality, can now be sustained, displaced, expressed symbolically, defended against. Its force comes from the built-in aggression potential in human beings, including its reactive forms, but its object, immediate source, mode of expression, and its sustained motivational character in itself, reflect developmental achievements. Thus, the status of an ongoing motivation is reached out of the reactive-aggressive potential and the human cognitive capacity to hold history and intent in mind. Here, too, as stated regarding sexuality, the aggressive drive not only is a part of the drive psychology but serves functions within all of the others as well. While oral biting, for example, has a prewired intimate tie to pleasure experiences, reactive aggression is stimulated by affronts to the ego's mastery (interferences with behavior) and to self experience (narsissistic injury), as well as by events within the context of early object relations that produce lasting rage and repetition.

CONCLUDING REMARKS

In his paper "On Motivation and Instinct Theory," Loewald (1971a) explored the development of "personal motivation." He writes:

Nevertheless [in the development of psychoanalytic theory over the years], motivation had become instinctual, as had repression and defense, in contrast to the early notion of personal will. Psychic life is motivated by sometimes conflicting, sometimes confluent, sometimes fused, sometimes defused, instinctual forces. There seems to be no room for *personal* motivation. Yet I have claimed that personal motivation is the fundamental assumption of psychoanalysis. We now seem to see that, on the contrary, psychoanalytic psychology postulates instinctual, unconscious, impersonal forces as the motives of our psychic life. Where is the person? Where is the ego or self that would be the source and mainstay of personal motivation?. . .

We are now prepared to give a preliminary answer to the question about personal motivation. Motivation, in the course of psychic organization, becomes increasingly personalized. The higher forms into which instinctual motivations become transformed and the more highly organized instinctual energy conformations which we call higher psychic structures, assume dominance to a greater or lesser degree within the developing individual. (pp. 110, 112)

But how has this come about?

Ego and id, conceived as psychic structures, come into being within the psychic unit the neonate is about to become by intricate interaction processes between conflicting, converging, and merging psychic energy currents surrounding and within the emerging psychic system; such interactions result in the organization of psychic structure. It cannot be stressed enough that *such organization is most vitally co-determined by the fact of the far higher complexity and organization of psychic energy obtaining in the (for the observer) surrounding or environmental psychic systems*. It is by the interaction with them that motivational forces of various orders of complexity and integration, and stable motivational structure of any kind, come into being within the newly emerging psychic unit, the child. On that basis, but *never without maintaining further interaction with psychic forces of the environment*, interactional processes within the new psychic system can be built into various forms of structural organization, whereby higher levels of motivation come about. (pp. 111–112) [Emphasis added.]

And yet,

instincts as the original motive forces never become extinct, nor do the structures corresponding more closely to those primitive forces. Thus the id is never superseded by the ego's increasing dominance, whereas the ego

may "regress," decrease in organization to a state closer to that level of psychic energy organization that we call id. It may be noted that the concepts
of sublimation and instinctualization and of controlled regression conform
to this picture of things. (pp. 112–113)

Thus, Loewald attempts to account for "higher" and more personalized
motivation via the development of the child in interaction with the environment which represents "far higher" complexity and organization. The end
result: an instinctual basis for motivation, but no slavery to "instinctual, unconscious, impersonal forces."

Sandler (1981) seeks to comprehend the wide array of differentiated personal "wishes" and "wished-for role-relationships" (all of which act as motives) in yet another way. As backdrop to his argument he tries to place
exaggerated uses of drive psychology in perspective. Thus, he writes:

Because psychoanalytic theory and practice has placed so much emphasis on sexual and aggressive wishes, and because psychoanalysis has
had to defend its findings in regard to the prevalence of such wishes,
there has been a tendency to see *all* wishes as instinctual. With developments in ego psychology after the war, psychoanalytic theoreticians
have gone through the most tremendous intellectual contortions to try
to derive *all* wishes from sexual and aggressive impulses, and have attempted to maintain a position in which any unconscious wish is seen
as being powered either by instinctual energy or by a desexualized or
neutralized form of that energy. (p. 187)

My aim in this chapter has been the same as that undertaken by the two
quoted theorists: to render an account of a wide array of individual motives
and to position them in relation to classical psychoanalytic theories of instinctual drive. The path I have taken is to show the developmental evolution of an array of motivations rooted, ultimately, in the biology of the
organism but *not* rooted ultimately only in that aspect of the biology of the
organism that is the source of instinctual drive. And, while the evolved motives that I have attempted to describe are conceived of as universals of development, it is certainly also the case (as I see it) that the "personal" forms
of these motives, in the term used by Loewald, take shape as products of in-

dividual history: the interactions with the environment and the adventitious circumstances of a particular life.

In this latter sense, once again, I want to say that my ultimate interest is in the *personal* psychologies of drive, ego, object relations, and self. There are formal theories extant regarding each of them. And there are arrays of phenomena to which these theories refer. But it is the personal form taken by these phenomena, including their individualized motivational quality and centrality, that are the real object of our interest, both developmentally and clinically.

In summary, then, I have attempted to describe ways in which phenomena in the domains of each of the four psychologies achieve clinically relevant motivational status during the course of development. In each domain there is present from birth a built-in, prewired motivational tendency, but these undergo developmental transformation; and it is the developmentally evolved motives that are worked with in the clinical situation. In the domain of object relations, we begin with a primal readiness for connection to the other and evolve tendencies to repeat old, now-internalized object relations in efforts at mastery of the strain trauma associated with them. In the domain of self experience, we begin with homeostatic tendencies to right subjective discomfort (the infant's cry when hungry), proceed through the development of familiar subjective states of self (self-constancy), and evolve a tendency to maintain that familiar self-state, though that state seen from the outside may be pathologically grandiose or abased, fragmented, or undifferentiated. In the domain of ego functioning, we begin with prewired capacities for responsiveness to stimuli and tendencies toward elementary reality attunement, tension regulation, and adaptedness, and evolve a (varyingly rigid, but never fully flexible) tendency to maintain the achieved mode of organization in an effort at avoiding negative affect. And in the domain of drive (both sexual and aggressive), we begin with biologically rooted urges which (a) become tied to specific objects and fantasies as those urges achieve cognitive representation and elaboration over time, (b) come to serve functions in relation to self experience, ego functioning, and object relations as well, and (c) in the case of aggression, come to include reactive forms which achieve ongoing status as the capacity to hold the offending other in mind matures (object constancy).

This recognition of an array of psychologically central motives raises the possibility that one or more of them can achieve dominance on the intrapsychic stage and lead to markedly different modes of organization of the personality. They speak for the possibility of a relative independence of motives governing various aspects of intrapsychic life. In light of this, and of all of the arguments and illustrations I have offered in support of the productiveness of a view from the standpoint of four psychologies, the question arises, how does the personality become organized so that the phenomena of each and all of the psychologies blend into the integrated (though conflicted) personality of each individual? Once again, in what follows, I shall approach this question from a developmental standpoint.

CHAPTER 6

Pathways to Personality Organization

HOW DO THE phenomena of the four psychologies get organized in the lives of individuals? That is the guiding question of this chapter. I shall attempt to answer it both developmentally (how the organization comes about over time) and descriptively (what such organizations may look like when we uncover them in psychoanalyses).

I shall build toward the conception that the phenomena of the four psychologies become organized in personal hierarchies, differing for each individual. The term *personal* reflects not only the view that they have their origins in unique individual life histories, but also that our theories and our concepts of health lead us to no specific, and certainly no unitary, conception of optimal outcome in regard to them. And the term *hierarchies* reflects the view that they get organized in *some* way, often with one or another set of phenomena being most central and putting their stamp on the rest. Nonetheless, clinical experience teaches that the hierarchies vary widely in degree of organization—from tight arrangements with one or more sets of phenomena central to looser arrangements with shifting centrality of issues.

It would be inconsistent with everything in this book up to this point to argue, say, that an organization around drive issues with adequate defense and sublimation, and with issues of self and object relations receding in importance, is automatically an optimal developmental outcome; or for a wholesome sense of self to put to rest "secondary" concerns with drive gratification. Either of these are caricatures. And a view of development (chapter 4) which sees critical early formations in each of the four areas, and life-span continued development in all of them as well, gives us no basis for championing the centrality of one or another set of issues as an optimal outcome.

These theoretical issues spill over into our concepts of mental health, which again turn out to be no sure guide. It may seem to be the case that excessive or monolithic domination of the personality by issues of just one of the psychologies is presumptive evidence of psychological disturbance. I have in mind such things as compulsive repetition of old object relationships as in the "fate neurosis," or preoccupation with maintenance of the integrity of a fragile ego defense system, or narcissistic self-aggrandizement, or an impulsive or repressive relation to some primary drive configuration. But these, too, are caricatures; no patient is summed up so simply. And, in any event, in my listing I am forced to picture not simply dominance by some particular issue in one or another of the psychologies, but also particular contents which are on their face pathological. And what of the other side of the equation—the golden mean as the model of psychological health? In this picture, issues of all of the psychologies are represented equally; no single one is dominant. But unfortunately this picture may characterize some chaotic personalities as well, wherein we see the equivalent of the polymorphous perverse personality—but here the polymorphous and nonorganized presence is not only of all of the psychosexual drives, but of unsettled issues in each of the four psychologies. I do not mean to be nihilistic on the question of mental health; only to say that I have no one-to-one relation to offer between the personal hierarchies and psychological well-being. The range of phenomena and the range of adaptations are both too wide.

INTRODUCTION: VARIABILITY AND STABILITY

Our theories seem to require concepts that help us account for stability, organization, "structure." Why is this? Shifting urges, moods, and environmental stimuli all make for variability. In my emphasis on moments of experience and function that are organized differently from one another, I start from a presumption of variability. And my whole emphasis on the four psychologies is intended to increase our recognition of diversity and variability in intrapsychic life, in development, and in the psychotherapeutic or psychoanalytic situation. Yet in adults, and even fairly early in childhood, much is stable, even somewhat predictable, in spite of variability. This stability had to have come about somehow in the course of development. The concept of structure is the one most often used in psychoanalytic theorizing to subsume those phenomena that make for stability and continuity over time. Structures as processes with a slow rate of change (Rapaport, 1960b) may capture something in terms of definition, but the concept really eludes definition. I shall stay with the somewhat softer terms *stability* or *organization*.

The movement toward stable organization is not linear over the life span. In fact, development itself is the greatest destabilizer, with new maturational forces (and sociocultural demands timed to them) upsetting one or another achieved order in intrapsychic life and, consequently, in behavior. Witness adolescence as a biological destabilizer of the school-age adaptation, or the entry into school (or into marriage or the work world or parenthood) as socioculturally derived potential destabilizers of whatever modes of adaptation had previously been settled upon. Nonetheless, there is a broad movement toward progressively more stable organization as development proceeds.

Numerous approaches to the description of progressive organization as a developmental achievement are explicit or implicit in the literature. I shall summarize a few of them briefly, as a steppingstone to my own formulations. None of these developmental views are inconsistent with any of the others; they all point to aspects of the movement toward stable organization. For the sake of explication, I shall group some of them under the headings "Transformative Organizations," "Cumulative Organizations," and "Committed Developmental Directions."

Transformative Organizations

The concept of the organizer as given by Spitz (1957) exemplifies such an organization. Something emerges in the course of development that both

reflects an achieved organization of prior developments and sets a future developmental course. After that emergence, personal functioning is never
again the same. For Spitz, the three significant early organizers are the smiling response, stranger anxiety, and the "no" response. Each reflects prior
maturation and learning, and each, once present, alters the infant's subsequent functioning in important ways. Thus, stranger anxiety is preceded by
the development of the infant's ability (a) to discriminate mother from others perceptually, (b) to "understand" that satisfaction and safety are linked to
the specific mother, and (c) to anticipate discomfort and nonsatisfaction in
mother's absence. These become interrelated with one another at about age
eight months to produce the newly emerging behavior patterns of stranger
anxiety and separation anxiety. With the emergence of these new behaviors,
there is a major thrust in the development of the specificity of the infant-
mother attachment that shapes the lines of their relationship thenceforth. A
mini-organization has taken place that is transformative in its effect, here on
object relation and on the modes of sought after gratification; defense, too,
in its anaclitic form, is affected, as the infant "leans upon" the mother's presence to stabilize his or her inner state.

For Mahler (1972), the rapprochement crisis and its resolution consti-
tute such an organizer. The rapprochement crisis reflects the coming
together of the child's opposing wishes for merger and for autonomy
with the recognized but at times rejected awareness of the mother's separateness. Its resolution is marked by the replacement of merger by object relationship, of primarily proximal contact by primarily verbal
contact, and by the move toward libidinal object constancy with the
mother carried inside. Again the emergence of the functional centrality
of these new phenomena radically alters the life course thereafter. Earlier
(Pine, 1979a), I attempted to describe the emergence of certain
affects—such as signal anxiety, longing, and guilt—as organizers in
Spitz's sense: reflecting prior developmental achievements (of which
they are the culmination) and altering the life course (regarding defense
functions, or attachments, or internal control, respectively) ever after. At
a considerably more abstract level within the classical analytic view, the
progressive differentiation of ego and id out of an undifferentiated stage
(Hartmann, 1939), and the consequent organization of mental life
around conflict (later added to by the development of the superego), is
another such transformative organization.

Cumulative Organizations

The concept of the representational world (Sandler and Rosenblatt, 1962) exemplifies cumulative organization. As experience accumulates in memory it gradually achieves representations that are not identical with any specific experience but that give an inner template for wishes toward and expectations of objects, an inner world of self-other relationships onto which actual relationships are in part mapped. Otto Kernberg's (1976) view that the building blocks of intrapsychic life are images of self and object bound together by an affect (that is, around an affectively significant interaction) is a parallel view, as is Leo Spiegel's (1959) discussion of the "pooling" of unfamiliar experiences (in adolescence) with old and familiar ones until the former, too, become a familiar part of self-feeling. All of these views describe a progressive (cumulative) build up of the images of inner life that together make for a certain stability of worldview: of self and other in relation or alone. None of this implies inflexibility to future change; yet it all bears on progressive developmental stabilization. So too do the cumulative effects of multiple identifications; such identifications gradually flesh out the "I," defining "who I am" with a certain degree of permanence. Each of these phenomena is part of a progressive organization of inner life which assimilates subsequent experiences to itself, influencing how they will be understood. Thus, gratification and nonsatisfaction in the inner world will each color, in different ways, the way the world of new experiences is "seen."

Multiple function (Waelder, 1936) can be viewed similarly. As significant behaviors come to accumulate additional meanings (Pine, 1970)—that is, to serve a wider and wider array of functions—they become more resistant to change. Each of these concepts reflects an attempt to describe the way sameness and order are achieved cumulatively in an individual life characterized by diversity and change.

Committed Developmental Directions

These views on committed developmental directions can all be described as variants on Robert Frost's poem "The Road Not Taken" (1971), in which he describes coming to two divergent paths, following one, and knowing that the further he follows its byways the less likely he is to return to follow the other. That is, they state that any life path we follow narrows our later choices by precluding other directions. At a psychological level, Freud's

(1916) views on fixation exemplify this. An individual with too much of himself or herself stuck at an early, say, oral or anal phase has fewer resources to move ahead to subsequent stages and more propensity to regression to the point of fixation. The life choice, here the fact of fixation, limits and alters all subsequent possibilities. If a child were constructing a tower of blocks, the size and stability of placement of each lower block would determine how high the tower could get without tumbling. History is inescapable. One can view Erikson's various dualities in the life span as capturing a similar set of epigenetically unfolding choices, each of which colors and limits all subsequent ones. Thus, the child who completes his earliest months with a sense of basic trust approaches the issues of the next phase (autonomy versus shame and doubt) with different opportunities for resolution than a child filled with distrust; and, for example, much later, in dealing with intimacy versus isolation, the issues of young adulthood, the opportunities of these same two children are again likely to be different. In these views, personality organization is a matter of progressive commitment, each developmental choice narrowing the degrees of freedom subsequently available. Some years ago I saw a mother and her preadolescent psychotic son in consultation, the two bound together in a symbiotic knot that the mother appeared to have fostered all through his early years as a way of dealing with her own aloneness. Now, as he was getting more demanding and more sexual, she wished (with one side of herself) to extricate herself. She said to me: "I can't wait until he becomes twenty-one and gets a job and gets married so he'll leave me alone"—this, as though the future choices were not already limited by the earlier ones.

Each of the views that I have been describing seeks to capture ways in which built-in aspects of the developmental process necessarily limit variability and/or foster a degree of stable organization. I should like to add another aspect of this process, one specifically directed to the progressive interrelatedness and individually characteristic organizations of the phenomena of the four psychologies. But first I want to address one theoretical by-product of the tendency for phenomena to come together in various networks of interrelatedness during the course of development. To do this, I return to the proposition advanced by Greenberg and Mitchell (1983) that mixed theoretical models need some conceptual glue to hold them together. They were speaking with specific reference to drive and relational models, but their proposition is certainly meant to apply to the even more mixed

model that I have been presenting here. Yet I contend that no conceptual
glue is necessary to hold them together; rather, development itself provides
the glue. It is not at the level of metatheory that we need look to bind together the person as seen from the perspectives of drive, ego, object relations, and self experience. Rather, we need concepts nearer to experience to
give us the language for describing the natural development of intercon-
nectedness during development. Baldly put, the linking of the phenomena
of these several psychologies is not a conceptual task but a developmental
event. I shall now go on to describe what I see as this event in three steps:
an expanded delineation of moments of experience, an argument regarding
the interconnection of those moments in terms of the evolution of multiple function, and a statement regarding their larger organization within
personal hierarchies.

MOMENTS

Winnicott (1963a) discussed the infant's "two mothers:" the "object
mother" who is the recipient of the infant's id tensions and the "environment mother" who protects, manages, and more quietly satisfies. One is a
drive object; the other provides a background of safety. This is Winnicott's
way of referring to divergent infant-mother experiences that occur at different times, dependent upon the inner state of the infant during the experience. Such different experiences will have different formative effects for
different aspects of the person.

I refer to such differences as moments—varying moments of varying
kinds of experience. The value of the emphasis on moments is to make clear
that there is plenty of time in the infant's day for experience to be organized
in the divergent ways addressed by each of the four psychologies. The young
infant is neither all oral (hungry and mouth-oriented), nor all symbiotic
(without differentiated self), nor all exploratory and perceptually receptive,
nor all object seeking. The infant is all of those things, at different times.
This view is not simply another way of naming the concept of state—for example, alert and receptive, vigorously crying, drowsy, or sleeping. Phenomena relevant to each of the psychologies can occur in the alert state or in
others. Let me illustrate some of these moments, and their relation to the
different psychologies.

The hungry infant awakens crying. The mother feeds her and the hunger is sated; quiescence returns. This moment in the life of the infant, repeated often, shows us the "conceptual baby" of the drive psychology—the baby on which the theory is built. Of course, much more is required and is represented in the drive psychology. There is a place for nonsatisfaction of the need and for satisfaction interlaced with maternal tension. There is a central place for the psychic representation of the biological need; for the child's wanting the mother and not merely food intake; and for the development of displaced, differentiated, mutually contradictory, and conflicted wishes and fantasies around such need states. And there is recognition of other bodily based satisfactions, involving anal or genital stimulation, and not only the mouth—as well as looking and being looked at, and causing and receiving pain—which at times has a pleasure component, and the psychic representations and convolutions of all of these. And aggressive urges and their expression and conflict over them are represented as well.

But the point is that the drive psychology, and each of the other psychologies, highlights one or another particular moment in the life of the infant, a moment consistent with its particular conceptual model—the conceptual baby required by the theory. I am of course not speaking of literal moments, but of states of experience that have some unitary character—they have a beginning and an end, and things are different before the beginning and after the end. They may be brief or of some duration; they may be quiet or they may be intense; they may fade slowly or end abruptly. But there is an experience that the baby is having (hunger, attentiveness, mutual cooing with mother, falling asleep at the breast, and so on) that begins to lay down particular memories at some point.

Each of the psychologies points to its conceptual baby, the moments in the life of the baby required by its theory. An ego psychology can point to visual tracking as a primitive reality attunement, to the finding of the thumb for sucking as a primitive adaptation, to a sinking into sleep in the face of nonsatisfaction or excessive stimulation as a primitive defense. An object relations psychology can point to early imitative facial expressions in the infant during face-to-face mother-infant play, or the infant's adaptation to the mother's rhythm or style—early forms of the infant's taking in and somehow carrying within the experienced relationship with the other. And a psychology of self experience can point, say, to the inferred experience of boundarylessness (Pine, 1986b) as the drowsy infant melts into the mother's body following feeding or, on the other hand, to moments of giddy pleasure (establishing a positive inner affect tone) responsive to the mother's own responsive, smiling, mirroring of the infant's behavior.

But all of these represent not only the conceptual babies of different theories but aspects of the real baby. These are moments in the lives of every infant, and there is every reason to believe that each is formative for different themes in the psychology of the individual. The infant is never a unity in terms of experience more than momentarily. In the oral phase the infant is not "all oral" any more than any infant or child is "all symbiotic" or "all anal" or "all oedipal" in those respective phases. Phases should not be conceived of as a time of life when the infant is continually one particular way. If this were so, how would we understand the one- to two-year-old's being in the anal, the separation-individuation, and the gender-identity-formation phases simultaneously? In recognition of the momentaryness of experience (that is, its varying psychological shape at varying times), I suggest that a phase be defined as the time of life when the critical formative events in respect to any particular area of human functioning take place. But these formative events can be based on significant *moments* of experience (in my example, involving anality, separation-individuation, or gender identity), and more than one can be taking place in any year, or half year, or even day or hour.

In sum, the infant has moments of many different kinds of experience, and these are formative for those diverse themes of personal functioning that are addressed by one or another or several of the psychologies of drive, ego, object relations, and self experience. Development, like all of life, consists of an endless sequence of such moments, at least some of which have a primary inner experiential organization that we try to capture with one or another of our various concepts. It is through such experiences that each individual begins to develop his or her *personal* drive, ego, object relations, and self psychologies. Our theories may or may not accurately reflect what goes on in the person in those several domains, but there are phenomena particular to each of them, and inner experience is built on and around these phenomena—hence the personal psychology, whatever the status of a particular theoretical psychology may be.

THE INTEGRATION AND ELABORATION OF MOMENTS

It is not necessary for my argument that "drive moments" or "ego moments," and so on, be seen as pure—that is, as involving phenomena addressed by only one of the four psychologies. That point was made only to illustrate that there are moments when different phenomena are central. Such moments are picked up by one or another theory as evidence for its perspective. But in fact, quite the reverse is the argument I wish to make. That is, no significant psychological phenomena remain encapsulated, untouched by everything else that is going on. Just as symptoms or character traits will accumulate new meanings, be invested with new fantasies over time, so too will the experiences recorded in these early formative moments.

Thus the situation of the hungry infant, waking, crying, sucking to satiation, and falling asleep at the breast, is central to the formation of the personal and unique drive psychology of the individual. The patterning of drive and its satisfaction begins to be molded at these moments through particular associated bodily/sensual experiences (touching, rocking, warmth) and through the pace and reliability of, or the intrusions upon, this satisfaction. But later, and certainly well within the infant's first year, with the infant more wakeful after feeding or capable of quiet delay before and during feeding, the nursing moment also comes to be a time of hand exploration of the mother's face, of mutually responsive cooing, of smiling, with all the implications these have for the development of the child's personal ego psychology—here, use and control of motor and vocal behavior, exploration, social adaptation, and defense (delay) itself. Additionally, and probably from the instant of the first mother-infant contact, vague self/object/affect experiences begin to be laid down, the core of the personal and internal object relations psychology. Or let us take the emergence of the "no" gesture and word (Spitz, 1957) as a core phenomenon in the personal ego psychology, promoting control and mastery. Inevitably it affects the object, whose altered responses (empathic or intrusive), together with the inner state of the infant at the time, will alter the object representations that are laid down and that become part of the individual's personal and internal object relations psychology as well. And, for example, the control the "no" gives to the timing and to the selectivity of object of drive gratification ("no, not now"; "no, this—not that") reshapes the personal drive psychology. Or, in the domain of initial self and object moments, the times of quiet mother-infant play, outside the press of need tension, are simultaneously formative for benign and loving object and self images and for the exercise of ego skills; additionally, these moments later (one could say early on as well) become involved in wish, fantasy, conflict—the world of more intense drive gratification.

All behaviors eventually come to have multiple functions for the individual (Waelder, 1936) and thereafter can be seen from the perspectives of each of the psychologies. Thus, to take an example easily at hand, the writing of professional papers has, for me, significant links to drive gratification, ego functioning, object relations, and self experience, and can be seen from the perspective of each of those psychologies. And if it did not have those functions initially, as paper writing continued to be an important aspect of my life, it would accumulate those functions as significant parts of my inner life attached themselves to this activity—just as they enter into my other work, my relationships, my vacations and avocations, and wherever. But it is not only obviously significant aspects of a life—like writing papers, or seeing patients, or relating to close family—that have these multiple functions, but less obvious things as well: walking, drinking coffee, reading a newspaper. Each of these, when significant to the individual, will have a particular history and a place in the personal drive and ego and object relations and self psychologies, and can be addressed from the conceptual perspective of those same four psychologies. This is true for each of us.

I began by stating that I have found each of the diverse conceptual perspectives current in the psychoanalytic literature useful in my clinical work. And I have been asking, how can there be a place for these diverse and perhaps even contradictory psychologies in the lives of individuals? My answer thus far has been to suggest that there are moments in the lives of every infant and child that are particularly formative for the phenomena addressed in the perspectives of each of the psychologies. If I give each psychology its due, it is because each deserves its due; in moments, there is time for all of them. But any phenomenon thus taking shape in the child gets interlaced with all the other phenomena taking shape in that same child. Multiple function becomes the rule, and any particular psychic event will, to varying degrees, ultimately be linked to the person's urges and wishes, ego functioning, object relations, and self experience.

Thus, the evolution of multiple function is crucial. New behavior does not spring forth fully formed, like Athena from Zeus's brow, with all its multiplicity of potential functions already in place. These are accumulated over time, as affectively significant intrapsychic/behavioral events attract new fantasies, become embedded in relationships, become central to the experience of self. So with the recognition of the growth of multiple function in this way, we can see how even the relatively discrete phenomena of specific early moments come to be elaborated upon and integrated with other phenomena, producing the complexity of thought and behavior that we try to unravel with the patient on the couch.

Other writers have given recognition to such processes of developmental linking. Phyllis Greenacre (1958), noting correspondences between speech and thought on the one hand and bowel control on the other (clean and dirty thoughts, verbal diarrhea or verbal constipation, orderliness or messiness in thought), points out that language development, early on, is taking place at the same time as toilet training; and she suggests that such co-occurring developments put their mark on one another. Thus, it is all one mind that integrates the co-occurring ideas regarding toilet training and speech, so the concepts regarding the one can readily spill over to the other. Through this, the (ego) achievement of speech develops meanings within the drive psychology. And Erik Erikson's (1950) work on zones and modes illustrates the same point—for example, the passive intake of the oral zone finds its parallel in the passive intake in the perceptual receptors, looking thus taking on an oral (drive) significance.

And the increasing complexity of particular moments of experience is added to from sources in the surround as well. Some time ago (Pine, 1982), I discussed the concept of appeal, as in "It appeals to me." What this experience reflects is our differential receptivity to environmental offerings based on their fit with our inner state. This is the appeal. In this way, specific inner experiences act like magnets, pulling in and incorporating those confirming and elaborating offerings from the surround that then add to and enrich the inner phenomena of particular moments of experience. Here, too, new meanings are added on.

But by far the most significant of the ways through which momentary experiences become elaborated and get pulled into central roles in the developing child's functioning is when the child's moments meet the mother's character and central fantasies. That is, what is a moment for a child will, in specific areas, varying from one mother-child pair to another, interact with what is a central area of conflict or failure for a particular mother (or other caretaker) with major consequences for its subsequent elaboration. Thus, an orally constricted or a self-indulgent mother will respond differently, in all likelihood, to the child's sucking moments than will a mother more at peace with issues of oral intake, giving those moments of the child's experience a differential shape—in its conflictful status or its centrality in the tie to the mother. And mothers with differing degrees of achieved individuation or conflict over symbiotic longings will respond differently to the moments of "melting" into the mother's body or the moments of autonomy in the child (see Mahler, Pine, and Bergman, 1970), with potentially fatefully different consequences for the child. And so too for all moments that meet or clash with the unique psychology of the particular caretaker.

But with this recognition of the significance of those moments of infant experience which come to interlock with specific conflictual or wishful or phobically avoided aspects of the caretaker's character and history, I begin to move beyond the issue of increasing psychological interrelatedness of moments and into the sphere of the rise of some moments to greater psychic consequence than others. Here we get into the establishment of the personal hierarchies, to which I now turn.

PERSONAL HIERARCHIES

The linkages that I have been describing, as multiple function comes to characterize all of our significant behaviors, represent a micro-organization of the phenomena of the several psychologies—this compared with the macro-organization that characterizes an individual's personality as a whole. It is at this latter level where we most often recognize the predictable sameness of one or another person. So, then, in what larger patterns do the varying phenomena of human function and motivation get organized? And what contributes to greater centrality for one or another aspect of that functioning and motivation? I do not mean to propose that with the development of multiple function everything becomes homogenized, a blur in which we all look the same, with a bit of this and a bit of that in all behaviors—these bits being the phenomena of drive, ego, object relations, and self in random array. Rather, I suggest that we each develop highly individualized personal organizations of these phenomena—we each develop personal hierarchies of the phenomena and motives of the four psychologies.

I can make my point clearer by reference to Freud's (1905) discussion of the eventual organization of pregenital sexual impulses around genital primacy. That is, oral, anal, exhibitionistic and voyeuristic, sadistic and masochistic urges—to degrees varying from individual to individual—find their place in foreplay, en route to heterosexual intercourse. Here is a model, within the drive psychology, for the organization and hierarchical subordination of significant psychological phenomena. A parallel model nicely captures what happens developmentally among the sets of phenomena addressed by the four psychologies. One or another becomes central and the others are organized around it. But which one becomes central in the personal hierarchical organization of the individual will vary from person to person. It is as though, in Freud's genital primacy model, genital sex did not always achieve primacy, but sometimes orality, or sadomasochism, or whichever. But, of course, that *is* the case, and under certain circumstances we think of such outcomes as perversions. It is certainly the case that varying ones of the four psychologies become hierarchically superordinate in varying individuals. But here there is nothing perverse about it. It just represents human variability. There can be greater or lesser pathology within any of the hierarchical arrangements, but health or pathology are not automatic consequences of the centrality of one or another set of issues.

Thus, I am suggesting three ways of looking at the interrelations among the phenomena addressed by the four psychologies. First, there are moments that, in relatively pure form, embody the issues of one or another of the psychologies alone—the hungry neonate sucking, the infant doing visual tracking during alert inactivity (Wolff, 1959); such moments are largely confined to the earliest days of life. Second, starting early on, and omnipresent in adult life (and already in childhood), is the development of multiple function: the intertwining of drive, ego, object relations, and self phenomena such that they each appear in all significant aspects of a person's functioning, describable from the perspective now of drive, now of object relations, now of ego function, now of self experience. And third, but in no way displacing the second, the phenomena of the several psychologies get organized, differently for each person, in personal hierarchies which represent relationships of super- and subordination among the phenomena of the

several psychologies. The idea of a personal hierarchy is meant to emphasize that no one of the psychologies has epigenetic (or theoretical) primacy.
For one individual, drive issues are predominant and others are organized in
relation to them; in others, issues of self-differentiation, or self-esteem, or
ego deficit, or the repetition of old internalized object relations. Our diagnostic thinking reflects such hierarchical arrangements; reference to neurosis or to narcissistic character disorder, for example, reflect a differential
centrality of drive or self issues, respectively.

Although the centrality of drive versus self issues is indeed a central con-
tending notion in the current psychoanalytic literature, it is hard for me to
imagine a full centrality of issues involving the repetition of old object relations unless these are also intimately tied to drive or self issues, because that
repetition would have to be powered by the kinds of psychic pain that stem
from disturbances in those areas. And to give equal potential status to hierarchies organized around the issues of the personal ego psychology requires
consideration not only of the evolved motive in the area of ego function—
the maintenance of one's own organization in order to avoid negative
affect—but additionally recognition of (a) ego fragility (the chronically fragile patient, or the incipient schizophrenic, who is desperately trying to hold
onto a sense of inner control and organization) and (b) the motivational
power of the dreads, avoidances, and humiliations that are crucial in some
individuals as a response to their awareness of personal vulnerabilities (ego
defects) that have caused them psychic pain or narcissistic mortification.
With these provisos, the point in principle remains that differing ones of the
several psychologies can achieve centrality in the personal hierarchy, the
personal intrapsychic organization, of different individuals.

How might we conceive of the differential shapes of such hierarchies? In
chapter 8 I shall try to concretize a response to this question with clinical examples; but, for now, let us just play with some ideas and images. We can
think of flexible versus rigid hierarchical dominance, with a greater rigidity
of and degree of domination by one set of issues itself a possible indicator of
pathology. Or we can think of the several issues as thoroughly interwoven
like strands of a rope (Stone, 1986), such that we only see them all bound together, the final rope of personality organization appearing as one integrated
whole. But we can also think of looser and tighter organizations—ropes the
strands of which are more or less tightly bound. In looser organizations the
multiple functions of particular behaviors may not always be as clear, so that

drive, or ego, or other issues may seem to stand almost separately at times. The reverse may hold in tighter organizations—for example, Mr. E in chapter 8, whose self-esteem issues put their stamp on all aspects of drive and defense as these emerged in the analysis. Or one can think of shifting structures—like in the game of cat's cradle, wherein a string can be shifted into different patterns, but is always returnable from one to any other. In this regard I think of my earlier (Pine, 1974) description of "shifting levels of ego organization" (itself an idea growing out of Rudolf Ekstein and Judith Wallerstein's [1954] work) in borderline children, here describing changing patterns within the ego domain itself—having to do with the overall level of defensive organization. What follows from this image is that one or another organization may be central at different times (see Mr. G in chapter 8), with the other(s) always ready to reemerge. One or another of these images may help us envision the diversity of the realm of personality organization built around arrangements among phenomena of the four psychologies.

How is the choice of the individual's specific personal organization determined? There are no general answers. The personal hierarchies evolve out of the accidents of personal endowment and personal history, in the endlessly individualized ways that we learn about and infer from patients on the couch. We are in the position Freud (1920b) was in when he viewed what we could know retrospectively versus prospectively. Retrospectively in an analysis, he said, the life story appears fully intertwined, as though the personal history could have produced no other end product than this particular individual. We understand how he or she came to this point. But prospectively, things are too open. We do not know, he said, the relative strengths of different psychological features; nor, I would add, do we know the future influential happenings. Without knowledge of these, our capacity for prediction is limited.

But there are a few general points worth making. Adventitious circumstances—such as the loss of a parent, major illness or multiple surgery, the presence of some actual defect—may play major roles in leading to the emergence of one or another issue as central in the personal hierarchy. But even here we cannot be sure which issue it will be; for even the impact of such major life facts will vary (in relation to drive, ego, object relation, self), depending upon the soil (the prior personality organization) in which they get rooted. Perhaps our best potential predictor of which issues will become central—though again this is limited—is the personalities of the primary caretakers. For when the child's moment meets the anxieties, seductions, or deprivations of the caretakers' character and conflicts the mix may be right for underlining certain experiences in such a way that they become central. Generational continuity is thus, to a degree, assured.

CONCLUDING REMARKS

I have attempted to propose a model for the understanding of personality organization across the four psychologies, based upon the development of personal hierarchies that establish which issues are superordinate and which subordinate. I wish to make three final brief points.

First, we have all been struck, in reading the literature, with how particular analysts seem to get from their patients material that fits with the analyst's own theories regarding mental life. Certainly we have all asked how much this represents a special sensitivity to particular material and how much it represents a biased shaping of the material. In the light of what I have written here, another view is possible—namely, that the analyst has picked up relevant content that is true to the patient (since all the issues are in all of us to some degree) but may have distorted its place in the personal hierarchy, building the analysis around the "found" content though it may have been subordinate to other issues.

Second, the multimodel view I have been taking can be seen as employing different perspectives on phenomena or as entailing the conceptualization of four overlapping but nonetheless relatively independent psychologies. I would propose that that distinction itself can profitably be viewed in developmental terms, and that there is a basis for thinking of the four psychologies in both ways. Very early on in development, as described above, we can see moments in the life of the infant wherein experience seems (from the outside) to be describable primarily in the terms of one or another of the psychologies. But gradually, as organization becomes more complex and behaviors come to have multiple functions, the phenomena addressed by the several psychologies become intertwined, and we are more likely to think of behavior now from this perspective and now from that, recognizing that phenomena of urge, of adaptation, of object relations, and of self are all reflected in anything the person does. Notwithstanding this development,

however, and also not canceling it out, as development proceeds and new
central motives are achieved in each domain, individual personalities get organized in particular ways that, now at a higher organizational level (rather
than in the momentary experiences of the infant), reflect a relative primacy
of one or another of the psychologies; at this point, once again, as very early
on, it may be useful to think in terms of relatively independent psychologies
—actually particular but widely differing intrapsychic dominance by one or
another—seen in one or another person. Like Spitz's (1957) "organizers,"
the later reemergence of relatively independent psychologies in particular
individuals can be seen both as a reflection of a developmental achievement
and as a marker of a future developmental course.

Finally, I do not mean to suggest that the establishment of any particular
set of issues as the dominant one in the personal hierarchy is more or less
"healthy" than any other. There is plenty of room for relatively better
adapted or more pathological variants within each of the domains. I refer to
them as personal hierarchies in order to emphasize the point that no specific
one is the natural end point of the epigenetic development of human beings. It may be that some idea of balance—that is, of significance of issues in
all of the domains, plus shifts in their centrality such that one or another is
more central at different times—would appear to be a recipe for mental
health. But that same description (significance of all issues and shifting centrality) can apply to chaotic and disorganized states as well. There is no substitute for evaluation and understanding of individual history and individual
function, and I turn to that in part II.

PART II

CLINICAL

THIS PART IS built entirely around discussions of clinical examples drawn from my own practice. The examples are intended to illustrate the ideas offered in part I and to demonstrate their source—that is, the clinical phenomena that led to their formulation. Each of the examples given here is from a patient in psychoanalysis, using the couch; but I see no reason that the phenomena described could not apply to everyone. They simply become more clear with patients working well in an analysis. In all that follows, I do not mean to present some new kind of psychoanalytic work: quite the reverse. The ideas presented thus far sit well, I believe, with psychoanalysis as it is ordinarily carried out. It is that "ordinary" psychoanalytic work that I mean to describe and comment upon.

Chapter 7 is based on process notes of sessions with four different patients. I try to give a sense of the work as it is actually carried on, with all its blemishes and uncertainties, so that readers can judge for themselves. Process notes are best suited for such a task. Process notes have another advantage. They are well suited to illustrate the normal flow of formulations from those in the language of one of the psychologies to those in the language of another. For the most part, and for purposes of illustration, I have selected sessions that include such shifts. I do not mean to suggest that the analyst should make a self-conscious effort to interpret now in the language of one of the psychologies, now in that of another. These examples are all from work that was going on as I was preparing for or actually writing this book and, typically, it was only after the patient left that it occurred to me that a particular session was a good example of the kind of shift that I am seeking to illustrate; during the sessions, I would simply be working, atheoretically to the degree that I am able. Nor do I mean to suggest that these kinds of shifts show up in every session. In my experience they do not. Many a session involves a question or two, perhaps a minor interpretation to keep the process moving, perhaps even significant insight in some particular area. But, although the shifts among the psychologies are not all that frequent, they are extremely useful for illustrative purposes when they occur, highlighting the sharp differences in forms of understanding, and so I selected such sessions for presentation here. At points of significant understanding, I contend, what we understand and convey to the patient varies along lines captured by the distinctions among the four psychologies; and therefore a multimodel view along the general lines that I have been proposing is reasonably well suited to capture the way psychoanalytic work in fact goes on.

Chapter 8 presents summaries and overviews of completed analyses. As chapter 7 is intended to give the reader a concrete sense of how the languages of the four psychologies appear in the everyday work of analysis, chapter 8 is intended to demonstrate the place of phenomena of each of the psychologies in the lives (and in the analyses) of individuals. It is intended to demonstrate that all of the phenomena appear in each analysis and to illustrate differing personal hierarchies—degrees of organization and of centrality—of the various sets of clinical phenomena.

CHAPTER 7

Some Psychoanalytic Sessions

MS. A, A fifty-two-year-old unmarried woman for whom this was a second analysis, came into treatment this time because of dissatisfaction with her functioning in her professional work. She was a book editor for a small avant-garde publication and, though without formal training, had made a specialty of reviewing books linked to psychoanalysis. She had become quite knowledgeable about psychoanalysis and had even tried (unsuccessfully) to write some popular magazine articles on the subject. In spite of some degree of external recognition, this daughter of two fairly well-known figures in the world of arts and letters was internally aware of real deficiencies in her thinking style, her grasp of ideas, and her capacity to convey what it was she wished to convey. She tended to get lost in endless rumination and to lose the sense of her cognitive purpose; this was why her magazine writing attempts had been unsuccessful. For her, privately, this led to a deep-seated sense of personal deficiency and failure; she wanted, as she said, "to straighten this out for myself, whether anyone else is aware of it or not." Her

first analysis had taken place many years before at a time of conflict over heterosexual relationships, possible marriage plans, and related issues; she felt
that that analysis had been helpful, but that the current issues were not yet
clearly central for her and had not been touchèd in it. The sessions to be reported took place in the second year of her analysis, but I shall also give a
view of some of our earlier work to set the context.

The thinking style that plagued her first entered the analysis in relation to
a dream that she reported in the third month. In the dream, she said, "an
endless rope of shit was coming out of me. I panicked when I couldn't pinch
it off, end it." Her first association was clear and straightforward; she remembered a rope-swallowing trick that she had recently seen a magician perform.
But then, in the session, something happened to the quality of her thought
process and speech, and she began to spin out an endless array of associations, without pause, one spilling into the next. I pointed out the parallel to
the dream, the endless rope of shit now coming out of her mouth, and wondered whether this was like the ruminative thinking that plagued her in her
work. She agreed that it was, said it frightened her to see how it even came
into the analysis, and then immediately shifted to speak of her "endless" dependency on me, or on her friends. She said that she tends to feel disappointed that people are not fully enough available to her, and then told of a
childhood relationship "that I never told anyone about before," which (for
her, internally) illustrated the endless dependency. She now was afraid that
she was showing me the "sick side" of herself and that I'd give up on her.
She said that her endless thinking and her endless dependency felt like her
two main problems.

After the session, wondering why this had come into the analysis at this
point, I recalled that she had been experiencing powerful, but vague, yearn-
ings the day before. In light of the "rope" coming out of her lower parts in
the dream, I did recall that there had been prior indirect references to male-
female bodily issues. I wondered about the rope as penis, but to my mind
this did not fit with where the patient seemed currently to be. So I waited.

Much else happened, of course, but I will skip to two sessions a few
months later by way of showing the development of this particular material,
and to prepare for the material of the second year, which is my focus—
reflecting a partial shift in the central language of the analytic work.

Four months later, following other reported dreams which led to endless
floods of associations, and based on reported memories of a particular style

of relationship that she and her mother had had in her early childhood (feeling "like one" through the mother's "glowing" over the child's talking and the child's "bathing" in that glow), I was able to suggest that her dream tellings were her way of reaching out to me, of bathing in my glow. She agreed eagerly and added: "And dreams are perfect for that. You're an analyst. You'll love dreams. But," she added [alluding to prior work in which I had suggested that the flood of associations was meant to obscure understanding of the dream content] "it's not that I want to obscure the dream. It's that *telling* the dream is my perfection, my contact. That *is* me." She went on to say that her rumination in her work situation is a problem only because she is often supposed to meet a deadline. But it is not only a *problem* to her. It is also her *pleasure*, her wish for "total immersion" ("bathing") in ideas.

In a session one week later, these ideas developed further. She recalled the many times she had been angry at me. Now she realized, she said, that her anger was often because of what she supposed was a "virtue" in me—that is, that I didn't just let her feel "blended in" with me as she wished. I managed to keep my separateness. She recalled her sense of her own badness in her adolescence when she tried to pull herself out of her old relationship to her mother—"I had needed it so, and my mother seemed to also, that sense of unity between us." She felt guilty when she tried to pull herself out, as though she were hurting her mother. In this session she also recalled feeling "vagued out," unreal, not a person in her own right until age fourteen when she entered her new school. This was a school that she had often spoken of as having been very important to her "because they encouraged *real* thinking and conversation in their students," not the kind of talk that she had had with her mother.

Growing out of material like this, the analysis in the first year had been largely around self-other boundaries (though I had never used those words). The phrase "perfect communion" had become the way we described it, communion especially around play with ideas—so central, inevitably, to the analytic process. All good analytic work in sessions would be *heard* for its content but *experienced* as this perfect communion/play and would tend to gratify her in relation to the very thought problem that had brought her in the first place. Even the jointly used phrase "perfect communion" gave her (in the very fact of its shared usage) that sense of perfect communion. "Why change these wishes?" she often asked and challenged me to answer. They were pleasurable, and she could find her way (with me) to satisfying them. I persistently showed her their denied "dark underside": the price she paid in her dissatisfaction with her work life and her hate for what she sometimes felt was the "infantile" part of her. Links to her mother had been central. Her mother (as recalled) glowed over the patient's every thought and word, but the mother herself was recalled as being inarticulate. Nothing was put into words; everything was left vague. I, in contrast, she said, put things into words. That made a difference; that was what she liked about me in our first consultation. She still felt the communion pleasure with words, but somehow it was making a difference. (My use of words simultaneously gratified the wish for perfect communion and fostered differentiation.)

In the overall context of this work, and now entering the second year of analysis, she began to get restless and angry. This was a "one-issue analysis" (all about boundaries). "You're keeping me an infant." She wanted "to grow up, but you won't let me." At this time, she was trying to work out a new writing project for herself with another editor. She referred to him by his full first name, but I misheard and thought she had used the diminutive form (as though she had said Anthony and I heard Tony). When I repeated the name Tony in something I later said, it got her angry; but she did not know why. It made her feel certain that I knew him, but felt that that should not come as a surprise. He, like herself, had some editorial links to psychoanalytically relevant books; she knew that I published in the field; and so it seemed unsurprising to her that I should know him. (I didn't, actually.) Nonetheless it angered her.

But then, in subsequent sessions, the former content, so dominant as to lead to her complaint about a one-issue analysis, started to shift. In the next session her father began to appear as a significant figure for the first time. He was seen (she made clear in this session) as an intellectual; her experience of him was quite unlike her experience of her mother (who was in fact a painter and not good with words). She recalled trying to get close to him in her adolescence, but felt he turned her away. Now she thinks that she probably tried to get close to him in order to get away from her mother; that was just at the time (she recalled) when she had entered her new school and loved thinking in the more articulate ways that that school encouraged. She would want to talk to him, to spend time with him. But his characteristic response (as she recalled it here) was to say, more or less, "You're not old enough yet; you don't know about the world yet." I said, "He, like I, was not letting you grow up." She saw the connection, but went on. She recalled turning to books at that time, burying herself in the library. She now wondered whether this was her way to find words for things (as mother never used) and to "learn about the world" (something father said she didn't know about).

She paused, and broke off here. She now said that something was feeling wrong between us ever since I used the name Tony a week or so before. I asked her what came to mind about that now. Immediately, she said: "I couldn't have said this then, when you just used it, but I can see now that I'm talking about my father. He always used 'pull' to get me jobs; he knew everyone. It made me feel I couldn't do it on my own. When you used the familiar name, it was like you *were* my father; you knew Anthony; you really would get me the job through pull and keep me an infant."

Following this session, the material, for the first time, began to expand more richly (not just as passing mention) into sexual and bodily issues. She began to talk about aspects of her current sexual life and sexual history. Her body was "all important" to her. She loved it when she was thin. She felt like a young boy then, or perhaps a pretty female; she didn't known which. She elaborated on her conflicts about her body.

In the next session (the last I'll describe)—and recall that she was familiar with analytic concepts from her editing and writing—she began excitedly: "Everything fits together! It's amazing! It's all clear now! I'm either a boy without a penis or my body is like a penis. I'm a girl-penis." None of this had ever been said to her by me and, while it made some general sense as I listened, what I was hearing primarily was the global thinking again, suffused by excitement, the symptom that had been the center of her first year's analytic work, and her presenting problem to begin with. I listened, and her thoughts seemed to me to continue on this global, excited track, becoming both more grand and all-inclusive, and more vague and confusing. I pointed this out. I said: "It's as though you assume that I know exactly what you are talking about when you say 'everything is clear' and it 'all fits together.' We have a perfect communion again. I'm your mother once more."

She stopped in her tracks. Then, after a long pause, she went on more quietly. "When I get filled with ideas," she said, "it's like being pregnant. I'm full. I'm content." Then, pensively, a thought: "Could this be like having a mind-baby with my father? My mother had a baby with my father [her younger sister], but she sure messed her up." She paused, and I said: "So ideas are your and your father's baby, but you won't let yourself do any better than your mother. You mess *them* up too." She stopped speaking and then, reflectively, softly, as though to herself, she said: "This is for real, isn't it? I can't believe this is happening in my analysis [rather than the one issue of boundaries]. It makes me feel grown up." Though I did not interpret it then, I saw the "this is for real" not only as a work of insight but as a sign of a different relation to ideas. Ideas could be "real," that is, *true*, and not only a basis for *experiences*; they could be part of father's *world* and not only of experience with mother. In later sessions, these themes continued to evolve, but I shall stop here.

I deliberately selected this series of sessions, of course, because they graphically depict a shift in the central issues of the analytic work. The issues of the first year, both in the recalled life history and in the transference, the issues captured by the quest for "perfect communion," were issues well described in terms of that point where self-definition and object relations are themselves not well differentiated. "Bathing in the glow" of mother's (and analyst's) receiving of her communications, wishing for that state and feeling infantile because of it, seeking it and projecting responsibility for it onto analyst, seeking to break out of it yet guilty in so doing—and all of this tied to the quality of her thinking that had brought her into analysis—she went through the first year of treatment. But, with the Anthony/Tony incident, the father entered the analysis. He entered first as the patient's means of pulling herself away from mother (as Ralph Greenson [1967] and Robert Stoller [1968] describe in terms of "disidentification from mother"); but subsequently he entered in terms of wishes for the oedipal baby and self-punishment (messing up her ideas) for her rivalry with mother. This did not mark a sharp break between issues of self and maternal object relations, on the one hand, and of sexuality and oedipal object relations on the other. For *ideas*, the form of the "perfect" relation to mother and analyst-as-mother, became also the form of the sought after relation to father and of the "idea baby" itself. The perfect communion ideas, reflecting lingering (though conflicted) wishes for merger, seemed to have a primary role in the relation to mother, served as a defense against the only slowly emerging oedipal fantasies involving father, and put their stamp on the form of that oedipal relation itself.

Though I regard this as a particularly clear illustration of the utility of thinking in terms of the several psychologies in human functioning, I do not regard it as in any way special as analytic work. I believe something like it happens all the time, and an open-minded and careful look at any work will reveal such shifts. As I stated in the first part of this book, I recognize that arguments can be made to reduce phenomena like these to the terms of any one psychology (here, say, self, or object relations, or drive); but I see no gain in doing so. Indeed, conceptually, I believe we have far more flexibility and our theoretical formulations are less forced (remember Sandler's words quoted on p. 95) if we work with the multiple models that psychoanalysis has thus far generated. And as for this particular patient, in the material presented I do not believe that we went "deeper" or reached the "real" issues of the analysis when the oedipal issues around father opened up. Each of the issues is real; each runs deep; each returned in the analysis again and again; and each was central in the termination phase some four years later. And of course they are not "separate psychologies" for the patient; in her life they are intimately intertwined, as I believe the presented material demonstrates.

Ms. B, a forty-seven-year-old recently divorced college-level teacher of English literature, came seeking treatment when haunting feelings of inadequacy, which she recognized as a lifelong backdrop to her life, crystallized much more centrally in her dealings with a senior figure in the administration of her university. The incident was deeply troubling to her, and yet familiar enough for her to feel that she wanted to try to come to some better terms with it. She had had a previous period of psychotherapy, which she regarded as quite helpful, and so the move back into psychological treatment seemed natural to her. Hearing both the longevity and characterological rootedness of the problem, and noting as well the patient's capacity for self-expression and self-observation, I recommended analysis, to which she readily agreed.

A second part of the context of her seeking treatment had to do with her relationship with her mother. Both her recent divorce and the entry of her second (and youngest) son into college away from home, left her more alone and threw her back more intensely into a relationship with her now aging mother. Ms. B's father had died in her preschool years and she, as an only child, had been raised in an emotional hothouse atmosphere alone with her mother, who never remarried. The mother-of-childhood is remembered as depressed, angry, and—especially—extraordinarily intrusive. At the time, early in the analysis, when the sessions to be reported took place, no very full picture of this early mother, or the way the relationship to her had worked for Ms. B as a child, had yet become clear. In Ms. B's later years—in college, during her marriage—she had kept considerably more distance from her mother, and the relationship cooled down. Being thrown back into a relationship with her mother after the divorce, and entering analysis, the patient became much more involved with the old issues of their relationship—but was no more ready than in the cooling-down years to come close to them.

An aside before I go on to report a series of three sessions: Self Psychology has brought attention to the significance of "empathic failure" in analysis (Kohut, 1977; Goldberg, 1978). As it has become a continually reappearing clinical concept in the literature, I have come to see it more as a characteristic of *patients* than of *analysts*. I do not mean to negate the fact that a clumsy, insensitive, or heavy-handed statement by an analyst or therapist can be hurtful, and seriously so, to *any* patient—given a sufficient degree of insensitivity. This involves the commission of empathic failures. But within the context of reasonably tactful analytic work, it is only certain patients who respond with the experience of having been failed to what in other patients would be experienced as relatively small "misses" of where the patient was emotionally. This experience is then a very powerful one—a deep sense of wound, of psychological abandonment or callousness, which takes considerable time and sensitive work to heal. The work toward healing is itself, as I have seen it, a central part of the analytic work. That is, it does not simply heal a breach that then enables "the work" to go on, but is itself the form in which the tendency to *experience oneself as having been failed* gets worked on and ultimately understood and worked through.

Ms. B was such a patient. At the time of the sessions to be reported, I already knew that she was particularly sensitive to anything on my part that made her feel pushed or intruded upon. I was coming to understand that, at least in part, this mirrored aspects of the early experience of being intruded upon in the relationship with mother. I was not and am not now entirely clear about how to understand this. Should it be in Self Psychological terms, as a narcissistic character structure, the result of deficiencies in the early relationship to mother, now structuralized in an ongoing experience of fragility in the face of further wounds to the self? Or in ego and trauma terms, as a vulnerability to a particular kind of overwhelmedness when a particular spark (the experience of intrusion) ignited the experience of the earlier conflagration/trauma at the hands of the mother? In any event, the sessions to be reported were a turning point in the emergence of a new object relational aspect in a particular instance of empathic failure. Once again, I view this new aspect of understanding not as an "instead of" but as an "in addition to."

In the first of the three sessions to be reported, the patient came in late and, in an astonishingly calm and perhaps even faintly breezy style, told of a series of things that had, by chance, all gone wrong in her life since the day before. None of them was a tragedy, but together or even singly they would be quite upsetting to any one of us. First, her house was broken into the night before when she was at the theater with friends; some things that were rather precious to her were taken, and the house overall was left in a mess. Second, some course teaching assignments for the following semester had been communicated to her the previous day, and she had been given very unsatisfactory assignments—quite out of keeping with the way things had been done in the past; she suspected, but was not sure, that this might be the result of her recent run-in with the university administrator. And third, a meeting with her departmental chairperson had forced her to be quite late to this day's session, something about which she was usually self-critical; she wanted to be exactly on time.

The events *were* troubling, but this would never have been known from her surface affect alone. However, just as she wound up telling me about them, her voice began to crack with a quiet tearfulness (of a familiar kind that had occurred often in sessions). As though bounding away from this, she shifted gears. "But things aren't *that* bad," she said, and began to list some (quite minor) things that had gone well—as though to balance the scale. Gently, I thought, since I was quite aware of her tendency to feel intruded upon and wounded, I interrupted at a pause, noted her attempt to balance the "bad" with the "good," and asked whether she felt not entitled to her pain (an idea that had come up in prior sessions). But she dismissed offhand what I had said, and continued in an almost compulsive style to list the "good" parts of the balance. At another pause, I said (I thought in a quite supportive tone, although well aware that I was edging her toward the painful affect that was already present in the tearful cracking of her voice): "I notice how you are fleeing the upsetting events. Is there some sense that you'll fall into an abyss if you let yourself experience any of it? As though it's all too much for you?" She became silent, then more fully tearful. Then she rejected the idea of an "abyss" and argued that it made no sense to get into the upset; she had to cope with the events, and she could do it better if she kept all her self-control. She was again tearful. When the session ended, she averted her face as she left. I did not know whether it was in anger or to hide her tears.

The next day she came in furious at me. I was "just a goddamn shrink" and had no ideas who she was or where she was at. I intruded on her (she said) and I pushed her. I had no awareness of her need to cope in her own way. When she left the day before, she was stuck in traffic—and she spent the time cursing me up and down. She was enraged with me. She added (in a statement that she had often made before) that she knows she hates it when I'm silent, but when I speak as I did the day before, it's worse. My silence and my speaking are both no good.

This was the general tone of the session. She calmed at times, went off on other topics, then came back to her anger. I was relatively quiet, not seeing a useful way to intervene. I also had a somewhat puzzled feeling. I still had the sense that my intervention the day before had been gentle, even though it brought her in touch with her pain, and I was somewhat baffled by the storm I had unleashed. I was aware of some inner tendency to justify myself, to explain in some fashion that I meant well, but this seemed inappropriate in light of my general sense of bafflement, and so it seemed wiser to be moderately silent (with enough words so that I was not experienced as punitively withdrawing), to listen, and to wait.

In the next session, after a weekend break, the patient's mood as she came in was clearly different, back to her usual more friendly self. She picked up on the previous week's sessions immediately. "You know, when you pointed out my pain it was like telling me to be like my mother. She would get distraught over everything. I guess you were right—it was like an abyss—but I didn't like hearing it.

"I had a dream over the weekend. Actually there were lots of family events over the weekend and I think they are connected to the second part of the dream." She then told me in considerable detail about various phone calls and family gatherings that took place over the weekend. The center of the story as she told it was of all the eccentricities she came to be aware of in members of her father's side of the family. She concluded: "My God, I wonder if there can be a genetic basis for eccentricity! Even John [a close male cousin on her father's side] who appears so sane is really eccentric. I'll tell you the dream. In it, I was going to my office. It was not like my regular building. It had lots of machinery in it. When I got to my office, my former therapist [a woman] was there—or it was supposed to be my former therapist. Actually it was another woman who I spent some vacation time with in Mexico last winter. I told her that I couldn't see her anymore because I was in analysis now. Then suddenly the scene changed. I was being examined for some kind of a neurological defect—that's the part that's like those eccentricities in my father's side of the family. I wasn't able to give the right answers in the examination, but I got angry in the dream in order to hide the fact that I didn't know the answers so they wouldn't find any defect."

She paused, and then, somewhat grudgingly, continued: "I suppose you want me to say what comes to mind about the dream. The woman in the dream, who was supposed to be my therapist, was someone I really liked, but—I don't know why—it's like she's dropped out of my life. The same happened with my therapist. I really liked her, but now she's not in my life either. It seems strange. They were both part of my life and now they're not. I've thought of going to see my old therapist—just as a friend, kind of. Just to see her once. Oh! The machinery in the dream was all red and green. Like Christmas. I've been thinking of visiting her [the therapist] sometime before Christmas; it's been on my mind lately."

I then spoke for the first time in the session: "I wonder if there is a third woman who used to be part of your life and whom you're now dropping out of it 'because you're in analysis now.' That is your mother. So neither you nor I will see the 'genetic' eccentricities on *her* side of the family that you've 'inherited'—like getting distraught as she does. And to make sure I didn't see the defect, you got angry at me, too, like in the neurological exam in the dream."

Ms. B's response was immediate. "My mother was always angry. You don't know what she was like." (And she went on to tell me about her anger.) When she finished, I said: "So, on Thursday you felt I was telling you to be like your mother, and on Friday you showed me what she was like—angry, like you were at me."

She responded with more about her mother. This time her emphasis was on the fact that you could never tell what her mother would get angry at. "Anything I did was wrong." I replied: "And that's the experience you try to create in me. If I'm silent you don't like it, and if I speak you don't like it. Anything *I* do is wrong. I guess you're showing me what it was like to grow up as you."

Now Ms. B laughed, and continued in a good mood: "It was fun to be angry at you. When I got stuck in traffic after that session and was cursing at you, I was really entertaining myself. I knew what I was doing. I really enjoyed it." Then, more seriously: "But I always tried not to yell at my sons as they were growing up. I didn't want to be like her." And I said, as I ended the session: "And yet, I tell you to be distraught, to be like her."

What has happened here? The patient's sense of having been injured by me, her sense of vulnerability—something that had come up a number of times before—suddenly changed shape, perhaps because of the specific content involved or perhaps because of where we had moved in the analysis. The organization of the material around the patient's sense of a fragile and vulnerable self—or perhaps around (as we can also conceptualize it) an ego easily traumatized by unmasterable intrusive inputs—suddenly shifted. In its place what emerged was a series of enactments of old object relations and identifications. I was her mother, intruding on her (with my first intervention). But then she was her mother, both of them distraught, an identification she felt I was pushing her toward. And then she was her mother again, angry at me, but this time with me in her childhood place as the child for whom anything she did was wrong.

I want to say that all of these interpretations of the enactments of internalized object relations were compelling, to me and to the patient. The fit seemed right, and the patient worked with them productively. But again, as I have said about the material on Ms. A, the turn to this other view of what was going on in her did not involve the dropping away of issues of her vulnerable self. Those certainly returned again and again and were for a long time the most central issues. And it is also clear that these and other issues were all interrelated. But they are best addressed, I believe, now in the language of self, now of object relations and, in the given instance (though we did not focus on it interpretively in these sessions), in the language of aggressive urge as well. The flow from one to another occurs quite naturally in some sessions. It just is what analysis is, and it is captured better in the multiple languages of the several psychologies than in terms of any one alone.

Mr. C entered analysis in his early forties. Childless and unmarried, he had been in a series of relationships, each of long duration, and felt stuck in a repetitive pattern in them. He would meet a woman, feel attracted and aroused sexually with her, and begin an affair in a highly sexual relationship.

But after several months he would find himself critical and nitpicking with his lover, always losing his temper and becoming attacking and abusive; at the same time he was feeling, if not quite righteous, at least not guilty— feeling, rather, that this was perfectly acceptable behavior. While his anger was growing, the sexual relationship would also turn sour, and eventually he would lose interest altogether. The relationship did not end at that point but, rather, dragged on in an angry, sexless state for a long while before it eventually ended at the instigation of one or another of the partners. He saw this happening again in his current relationship, but this time was impelled to do something about it.

In the months prior to the session to be described, a number of understandings had been achieved in relation to his anger outside the sessions and a tendency toward "helpless" (stuck) silence in the sessions.

Taking the former first: The patient's father was remembered as dominating the household with his nasty and critical opinions about every family member—the patient, his two older sisters, and his mother. Home was experienced as a dreaded place. When patient was in school or with friends, he could be active and outgoing; but upon entering the home, even if his father was not yet home from work, the patient's behavior radically changed. He felt constrained and inhibited, already anticipating father's return, and he tried to stay silently off on his own. He remembered feeling absolutely worthless under the barbs of father's critical attacks on him, and he carried that feeling still. In innumerable sessions and via innumerable routes, his current angry and attacking behavior was seen in relation to his retention and reliving of that old traumatizing internalized object relationship. We came to see that, in his anger, he was being his father; it gave a peculiar kind of comfort; it was as though he was able to carry his whole family atmosphere with him through his life. It also felt very "normal"; the experience of his anger as "perfectly acceptable behavior" linked to its being the unquestioned and certainly unchallenged way his childhood household had run; this was just the way things were. And, of course, it turned the relationship from passive to active. He was not the criticized child; he was instead the criticizing father; furthermore he made his lover into his old self, the criticized child. This much seemed clear. The patient had two persistent reactions to it. The dominant one was a constant refrain: "I can see it's just like my father, but I can't stop it"—usually with an "I did it again last night" incident recounted. The other reaction, simultaneously, was a growing sense of ego alienness of the angry behavior and a feeling of pleasure at each restraint of it.

The second set of understandings in the months before the session to be described, understandings largely though not entirely in the same object relational context, had to do with the patient's feeling of helpless inarticulateness in the sessions. He was well aware of a certain contrast: with his lover he was vocal and critically attacking; but with me he found it hard to say anything. He believed that whatever he said would not be worth anything, and that eventually I would tire of him and terminate the analysis because he was so stuck. (In fact, though there were often long pauses, the patient could hardly be described as a silent patient; being silent and stuck was more an inner experience.) The interpretations that met thoughts closest to the patient's awareness, and with which he was most comfortable, also had to do with repetition of the old object relationship. He was in a knot: he was silent because, if he spoke, I (as father) would criticize him; but, turning full circle, if he were silent I (as analyst) would also criticize him and end the analysis. The silence, also, like his anger, re-created the atmosphere of his childhood home—keeping it alive for him; but here it re-created his own fearful withdrawals when he entered the home, exactly, he noted, as his behavior changed from expressive to blocked as he entered my office. An understanding of the silence that became strikingly clear, but that gave the patient more discomfort, was its role in sexuality; he was aware that a certain silent tendency when first entering a relationship with a new woman seemed to interest the woman in him; she would "fill the silence with sex," and he would feel that the relationship was off to a good start.

Except for this last point regarding sexuality, the achieved understandings of both the anger and the experience of helpless silence were largely in terms of the old family drama with his father, now internalized and carried into the present with the lover and with me. In the session to be described, an additional understanding rapidly emerged.

Mr. C came in for his session and immediately said that he had had a dream, but that he couldn't remember it. "It was something about fighting with Jane [his current lover], but it was vague." He then dropped it, and seemed to be searching his mind for another topic. After a pause he came up with one, as though managing to find another thing to say: "I was reading a novel last night. It's about these people and their sadomasochistic relationships. A lot of sex. It was as though the writer was telling us his own fantasies in his novel. I was amazed at how frank people could be about expressing their fantasies. I could never do that. . . . I used to have fantasies like that when I was younger, but not anymore. [Another long pause.] I'm blank. I don't have anything to talk about."

Occasionally in prior sessions I had commented on the blankness and silence in terms of Mr. C's withholding thoughts that he was in fact having. This had at times led to a ready opening up. But equally often it had seemed to miss the mark, and had led me to focus on the silence itself as the significant communication for the patient. This approach had led to the understandings about the place of silence in the patient's object relations. But in this current session, following the dropped references to the dream of fighting and to the sadomasochistic fantasies earlier in his life, I again addressed the defensive aspect of the silence. So, in reply to his "I'm blank; I don't have anything to talk about," I simply said, "I guess the dream and your old fantasies don't count."

The patient laughed, anxiously and self-consciously, and went on. "I don't know what to say about the dream; it was a fight again, like I'm always doing with Jane. . . . I used to have those [sadomasochistic] fantasies a lot. It went both ways. I'd be in the woman's power, tied up or whatever. She could do whatever she wanted with me. Or else I had her in my power. I could really dominate her, do whatever I wanted. That was the main way I had them. It was a real turn-on. I don't know what happened, but I don't have those fantasies anymore." After another pause I said: "Perhaps now they are lived out, in your fighting and attacking, but now with the sexual part not so evident." This produced the following exchange.

"But if that were so, shouldn't I get some pleasure in my fighting?"

"Are you ever aware of any?"

After a pause: "Yes, I am. I get flashes of pleasure, but I try to put it out of my mind; I don't like to think of it that way. In those fantasies I would really be at her mercy; or she would be at mine. I'd have her at my mercy and could do anything sexual I wanted. . . . [He continued, in an apparent non sequitur]: If you want to see it that way."

"Why do you add that last phrase?"

"Because you suggested that I should talk about the fantasy."

"Oh! I see. You're at *my* mercy here."

The patient immediately went on: "I felt at my father's mercy when he criticized me." He talked about this in some detail, giving a good sense of his being "at his father's mercy."

After a while there was again a pause and again Mr. C said he felt he didn't know what to say. But this time he picked up on his own blocked feeling. "I don't like what we're talking about; I can't stand all this focus on me. And I can't stand the silence. I guess I'm stuck either way. I don't see where . . . . It's like I play it out for a whole lifetime. I'm starting it here again. I'll get silent; I'll be at your mercy; you'll throw me out."

After another long pause, I said: "I wonder if that works both ways, too. Like you say, you're at my mercy; if you're silent I can throw you out. But silence is powerful. With it, *I'm* at *your* mercy too. What can I do if you are silent?"

Again the patient confirmed this readily: "You know, they say silence is deafening. It *is* powerful. Sometimes when I'm silent in a group everybody starts to focus on me. They don't know what I'm thinking, and they want to know. [Then again there was a non sequitur—and a form of statement not at all typical for this patient.] Is that what you wanted? Did I answer your question?"

Again I said: "So, again you're at my mercy; I have all the power." The patient picked up again and spoke for about ten minutes, until the end of the session. After an opening of, "God! I can see I do it over and over; either you have the power or I do," he went on to describe two things. The first had to do with the way his father was friendly and charming out of the home, but attacked him within it; the patient felt that his "flip flop" as he entered the sessions and became silent was somehow like that. Then he spoke of a phone conversation of the night before. In it, he felt he was giving good advice, but had been haunted during the conversation by the feeling that he was dominating the other person. "I kept thinking: 'Is this right? Should I keep my mouth shut?' I don't know when I'm overstepping myself." And here the session ended.

In this session, the use of silence to defend against the revelation of sadomasochistic fantasies, and the sadomasochistic aspect both of the silence itself and of his fighting, entered the treatment firmly and to stay, adding to (but not replacing) the view of both silence and fighting as a repetition of an earlier object relationship and serving various present-day functions. The patient was not comfortable with this new view and continued both to evade and to confirm it. What also began to enter the analysis after this point, in addition to the sadomasochistic fantasies themselves, was the central role of fantasizing as an activity in Mr. C's childhood life—something that the silent blankness served to reverse. Our view of his silence was now informed by the drive psychology (his sadomasochistic fantasies) and the object relations psychology (its place in repetition of old relationships). But the ego psychology (its use for defense), and psychology of self experience (as it was core to his sense of himself, deeply coloring his feeling of low self-esteem) were also part of the picture as we came to know it.

In this last, somewhat more complex, example, the material again flows in directions suggestive of all four of the psychologies.

Ms. D, a thirty-two-year-old married woman, had not been working since the birth of her twin girls four years earlier. She first came to see me when a serious illness in one of the twins produced great inner distress and then considerable difficulty (anger and loss of closeness) in the mother's relation to the other twin. She sought a consultation with me to discuss how best to cope with the dual problem she was encountering. Two things happened rather rapidly, however. First, it became apparent that Ms. D's tendency to feel overwhelmed by the situation, flooded with bouts of anticipatory grief, anxiety, and anger, were characteristics of her affect life of long standing. One thing or another had always easily triggered the feeling of being overwhelmed or flooded; the illness and conflict, respectively, with the twins was but the most recent triggering event. The second thing that happened was that the child's illness turned out to resolve rapidly, things returned to normal with the second child, and family life restabilized. The consultation ended. But about six months later Ms. D called me, seeking analysis for herself around the affect flooding. The treatment began soon afterward.

Ms. D had been raised in a suburban area in France, the second and last daughter of a couple that together ran a small family business. Her mother, active in church affairs, was a kind of informal social worker for the community. At home, however, the mother was experienced as being driven, depressed, and rageful, and there are reported instances of her actually losing control and becoming physically assaultive. The father, aside from his business, was a cycling enthusiast. He had twice raced in the renowned Tour de France, once coming out not far behind the victors. Both of his daughters seemed to have been encouraged to become excellent cyclists; but they also came to pursue that goal on their own, as a way of establishing a closer relationship to their father, largely based on satisfying him and winning his approval. The patient often felt insufficiently successful on the bicycle (by father's standards of form, endurance, and speed) but always resolutely returned to it and tried again. The father had also had dreams (never materialized) of emigrating to the United States, where two of his brothers lived, and in anticipation had arranged for each of his daughters to have tutoring in English from an early age. As a child, Ms. D had considerable difficulty with this. While her sister learned English well, she struggled painfully with only minimal success. The term *learning disabled* was not available to the family, but the child was nonetheless defined in that way informally; the sense that something was wrong with her head pervaded her growing up years. Years later, Ms. D came to the United States after meeting and eventually marrying an American whom she had met while he was a tourist in France. She speaks English well now, with a marked accent but with no sign of difficulty.

I shall summarize three sessions (and some of the surrounding material) that took place within a few weeks of each other, all shortly after the first summer break in the analysis. The issues in the three seem interrelated, but emerged in different perspectives during this time. In anticipation of that summer break, the patient had shown intense feelings of abandonment and rage. She described herself as being "overwhelmed," but she resolved to be absolutely competent during the summer so as not to give in to such feelings. In the first postsummer session, Ms. D was again flooded with the feelings of abandonment and rage.

In the first session to be described in detail, the second after the summer break, she came in under considerably better self-control, saying that she had the urge to make some offhand comment that would lightly dismiss the previous day's session. She could come up with none, but went on to say that one incident from the summer was sticking in her mind and she wanted to tell me about it.

"You're in this," she began. During the summer break, a friend who knew the patient was in analysis asked her how she had located the person she was seeing; the friend wanted to begin treatment also and was feeling some urgency about finding someone for September. It was a close friend, and the patient wanted to be helpful; she thought of asking me for a referral name, but did not want to call me during the summer break. So she decided to write to me, but the letter had come back "addressee unknown." It was not until leaving the office the day before, when she happened to note the address on my building, that she recalled the incident and realized that she had reversed some of the digits in the address. "What was that about?" she wondered aloud. The night before this session she had called to check with her friend about where things stood in his search for a therapist, only to learn that the friend was no longer interested; this enraged my patient.

But for the patient, in the telling, what was central (she said) was that she had wanted so much to be taken care of—and here she was, taking care of others. She became tearful. "I always do that." And just like *I* didn't take care of *her* (by leaving on vacation), she said, the friend didn't let her take care of him (by refusing the referral). "I wanted to be in touch with you, to make a contact [through the letter, but also by being competent—both planful and in control of her emotions]. I so wanted to be important . . . important to you." She went on about being important to me so that I wouldn't leave her. She wanted me to miss her as much as she missed me. The wish for the object tie seemed central in these thoughts.

At this point, about twenty minutes into the session, I spoke for the first time: "You said: 'I wanted to be important.' But then you added, 'Important to you.'" (I had heard that added "to you" as a kind of cover-up, which puzzled me.)

The patient immediately picked up on this. "When he didn't accept my referral, I felt *diminished*. I hate that feeling. You know, something else happened during the summer about being important. My parents were visiting from France and we all went out to take a family photo. I kind of wanted to be in the center, to take up most room, but then I felt troubled by this. It reminded me of an old family photo from childhood; I even dug it out afterwards to look at it. That night I had a dream. There was a family photo. I was very large, almost inflated, in the center of it. When I awoke I began feeling really troubled about the photo from the day before. I worried if I had hogged all the space. I didn't feel relieved until the photo was developed and I saw that I hadn't hogged any space; I wasn't even in the center."

She suddenly said: "I forgot the point of all of this. What was I talking about? . . . Oh! Something about being diminished." I was thinking that, with the "I wanted to be important" and the associations following it, we had shifted from her sense of object loss to her narcissistic wounds. I knew from prior work that the "learning disability" was a narcissistic injury to her, and that had made its appearance in this session with the miswritten address and even, I thought—again from prior work—in the momentary forgetting of what she had just been talking about. I wondered about the object loss—my vacation—"diminishing" her in the same sense as the learning disability had—that is, my going away was both a loss of a love object and a blow to self-esteem. But I chose not to say anything at this point both because the patient seemed to be working so well on her own and because, with what I knew of her mortification in this area and with the fact that the hurts of the summer break were still so raw, it seemed to me that it might be pushing too quickly, tactlessly.

But the patient, evidently on the same wavelength herself, went on to connect the "diminished" self-feeling to object-related issues. Without any intervention from me, and therefore directly following her recall of the fact that she had been talking about feeling diminished, she said: "If I feel diminished, I'm more worried about your criticism. How can I take you in [that is, carry me with her internally for the summer] if I'm not in the center, if you are critical of me instead? My father used to criticize me as though it were love. He'd say [when he criticized her when she had difficulty meeting his cycling standards]: 'I tell you these things because I love you.'" She added, as an aside, as though to herself or to her father: "If you loved me, you *wouldn't* say those things to me." Then she made a pause, a recovery, and as I ended the session she said, playfully: "I wanted to cut my hair shorter over the summer. That would 'diminish' me; but I thought it would make me cuter and more lovable."

Certainly not everything becomes clear here, though a lot is suggestive. Some of it is clearer to me, based on prior work; some becomes clear later on. But the flow of this good analytic process dips into different, and intersecting, regions of the patient's intrapsychic life: the obviously effective observer capacity and use of humor from the side of ego functioning, and yet the question of ego defect in affect control as well as the experience of being defective in relation to the learning problems; the issues of self-worth and esteem in relation to experienced defects, but also in response to being left by the object, and the compensatory grandiosity (being important, in the center), and the clear conflict over that; the struggle to contain and also to express both aggressive urges and dependent needs, both in turn related to the object loss; and (more speculatively, and not directly appearing in the context of this particular session) the whole object-related history with mother's rages, which seemed to provide a model, through identification and repetition, for the patient's "overwhelming" rage as well as, perhaps, one of the origins of defective early learning of affect control. All of these issues in the separable but intersecting domains of drive, ego, object relations, and self continue to find expression in the two further sessions that I shall summarize.

This next session follows by three the sessions just reported. In the intervening sessions the patient had continued to talk about her feelings of abandonment and rage. They fill her. Her rage feels endless, never ceasing. Her needs feel like a "bottomless pit." Her rage is also "lethal"—that is, it destroys the very relationships she is angry about not having. But through all of this her observer capacity is always present, and the therapeutic alliance is firm. The patient is clearly *telling* me of these experiences, not simply living them out—wanting to work on them with me to get out of what she feels to be a hopeless morass. Further aspects of her relation to her mother had come up in these sessions, clarifying much of what was going on—but not lessening the feeling of being overwhelmed from inside herself.

The session immediately preceding the one now to be reported had ended in such a way that I found myself with the thought: Was she right? Was her rage "endless" in some sense? Was there something defective in the internal control system? Were her needs "bottomless"? And what would such an idea even mean? Was there some early fault in mothering that produced such an effect? The questions floated through my mind. A second thought was left with me also at that time. She had ended with the idea: "I'll never be satisfied until I know I'm the most important person in your life," but she had said this with the pained sense that this was hopeless, foredoomed. It touched off, in my mind, remembrances of her relation to her father. With him, she had had that wish—to be the most important person to him—and had worked hard to win that position in his eyes.

The session I shall now describe began with her saying: "I wish I could bring some levity into this. I wish I could show you my good side." She hated coming in, lying down, and having her "bad side" take over. But, having said this, the rage/abandonment mood and content began to fill her again. She was saying that this always fills her and destroys her relationships. After about ten minutes, undoubtedly influenced by my thought after the previous session—were the neediness and rage "bottomless"?—I asked: "Was it ever different in any relationship?"

Almost without pause she said no, and then added that she felt I had tested her just now and that she had failed the test. But then she said: "Well, in fact, it was different" with her elder sister, Sue. She could talk to Sue, confide in her, get guidance from her, and generally count on her. "Sue was strong, like steel. In her character I mean. She would try anything, and do it. She was the boy my father had wanted." She went on to describe her sister's cycling feats. I had heard before, and again now, of the patient's endless efforts to be a strong cyclist, to go great distances, to have the proper form—but how she was never good enough for her father. But now I learned for the first time that her sister was always the expert and won some local cycling prizes. Sue was, along with their mother, "the most important person" in her father's life. But patient kept trying—by continually returning to her cycling and trying to get better at it—to meet his approval. And she added how she had also tried to woo him in other ways, which she then described.

At this juncture, about two-thirds of the way into the session, I made my second comment. She had often, and again recently, compared herself with my other patients, saying I couldn't possibly like her as a patient because she was so needy and rageful. So at this point I said: "Getting on the couch each day sounds like getting back on the bicycle. You'll keep trying to please me, but you know I like all my other patients more; they do analysis, bicycle riding, better than you." She responded, suddenly calm and thoughtful, "Yes, it feels just the same as getting on the bicycle." Then, after a thoughtful pause: "By anyone else's standards I was a good cyclist; but not by his. His standards were so high." I added: "As you imagine mine to be. So all my other patients are better than you. You can't show me your good side; no levity. I can only see the side that will be 'lethal' for the relationship." The patient responded with a long silence that seemed thoughtful.

After a while I broke the silence and said: "Your rage, and your sense of helplessness about it, and your neediness, often seem like things that *happen* to you. Like things that take over and fill you, overwhelm you. Like a needy child whose mother abandoned her emotionally, and whose needs and rage swamp her. But now it sounds like your hopeless rage is also something you *do*. You *keep* getting back on the couch, back on the bike, and you do it ragefully, because it feels hopeless. You feel you won't get what you want, yet you're going to keep trying, almost stubbornly, until you make it come out right this time, until you're the most important person in my life." She responded fairly quickly, with a smile in her voice: "Right! So now what am I supposed to do about it?" After a pause, I said, "For now, perhaps just think about it," and ended the session.

In retrospect I can see this session as a turning point. It was the first time that the feelings of being overwhelmed were considered, not only as a defect in the balance of drive and defense based in part on early identifications with the rageful mother, but as an insistent attempt at repetition of old relationships, to demonstrate again and again their inevitable failure but also to make them turn out better. (Later, when making them turn out better got to be seen as a possibility, it in turn produced anxiety and "overwhelming" excitement.) What had been introduced was the contrast of ego passivity (the rage "happens") versus ego activity (it is something she *does*)—a central issue for drive control and ego defense. These various themes came up again in particularly clear ways in a session a few weeks later, the last I shall summarize.

The day before, I had, dealing with the issue of her experience of feeling defective, made a fairly extended summary statement and a new formulation toward the end of the session. I had said: "I know you *feel* defective with respect to your learning difficulty as a child, and with your tendency to get overwhelmed by rage, and because you were born a girl when your parents wanted a boy [this had come up often]. And beyond that, I know you also believe you *are* defective."

"I am defective," she interjected, challenging me, "and what can we do about it?"

I went on: "But what you are not aware of is how much you put your sense of defect right smack into the center of your sense of yourself and live your life around it."

Again she responded, as after the previously summarized session, "So what am I supposed to do about that?"

On this day she came in and said: "I know you said a lot at the end of the session yesterday, but all I remember is that you said something is wrong with my mind" [thereby illustrating what I had said but not seeming to hear or understand or use it].

"Is that what I said?"

"Maybe that's what's wrong with my mind; I can find something critical in anything you say." She berated herself about this for a while, and then asked: "What *did* you say yesterday?"

I responded, "I don't mind repeating it, but why don't you go on for a while first?"

She immediately went on: "I feel I keep a balance in my life. They [her parents] always said I couldn't accomplish anything intellectual. But now I *am* accomplishing that and I want to say, 'See, I'm doing it!' And I want to keep the struggle going."

"That's pretty much what I said yesterday." (I repeated it briefly, focusing on the way she keeps the sense of defect central—here by "keeping the struggle going.")

She responded, now tearfully, plunging back into the sense of defect: "I feel that whatever I learn goes inside and falls into a deep hole. It's bottomless. It just falls inside and gets lost in there."

I asked: "Is that what your language disability was like?"

"No," she answered. "I had no trouble remembering. Just with grasping things in the first place."

I said: "From things you've told me, it sounds like you probably did have some kind of disability with learning as a child; but what you just said sounds more like a fantasy about your body. *You* are the bottomless pit—so needy that it's endless, and having no bottom because you're a girl [both things that had come up before, but not in connection with the learning disability]. It's as though you say, 'I can't learn because my mother didn't love me enough and because I'm not a boy'; and the 'disability' is paraded as proof."

The patient's tone changed; the observer in her came more to the fore. She became stronger, clearer. She told me in some detail about the way she fumbled and messed something up in a class recently—starting by misplacing her notes. She realized she was trying to prove to me that she was dumb, but then added: "*That* doesn't sound like a learning disability. It reminds me of copying the wrong address for that letter to you during the summer. It sounds more like anxiety. . . . I was enraged at that woman [her class instructor, in the just reported incident when patient misplaced her notes; but she was also enraged at her mother and probably at me during the summer break]. How can I think straight when I'm enraged?" She paused. I was silent. Then she went on, reflectively: "I was noticed in my family when I had trouble learning. That was my role. It was the only way I was special, the most important one."

I interjected; "Perhaps with me too—my poor, hopeless, defective patient. My special one."

She went on, half tearfully, half laughing at herself: "But if I tried to be smart I'd have to compete with [here she named some well-known female scholars] . . . and compete with you . . . and I'd never be noticed."

I replied, "So you can be a success at being a failure, but you'd be a failure at being a success."

She became silent. It was near the end of the hour, and she sensed that. She said: "Is time up? I want to leave." I asked what was going on inside her. She said: "I'm afraid to talk about my mother. I'm afraid I'll feel a horrible sense of longing." (This was the first time in over a year of analysis that the idea of longing, rather than rage and abandonment, came up in relation to mother.) The session ended.

The sessions just described occurred early in the second year of this analysis. They were clearly the beginning, not the end, of the work. Much more developed later, and many changes took place in the patient. But these sessions permit me to illustrate and discuss the multiple models of psychic functioning that are regularly revealed in analytic work. I shall highlight them in relation to two of the central issues: the experience of overwhelming rage and the learning disability.

The rage was productively seen in terms of defective (ego) control based on identification with the ragefully out-of-control mother. But additionally it was seen as a mode of continuing the enraged relation to the parents (analyst) in an effort simultaneously toward retaliation and toward mastery (healing); here the repetition of old internalized object relationships becomes central. She was going to make those relationships come out differently this time and also to prove that they would not—that the parents (analyst) were bad to her and deserved her rage. (Still later, not in the presented material, it emerged that the rage also served as a defense against sexual thoughts and urges, the one urge defending against—that is, replacing—the other.) As each of these became clear, stepwise in the course of the work, they did not replace the earlier views of the place of rage in her intrapsychic life. We did not come to see the rage as "really" a repetition of the object relations or a defense against sexuality, say, rather than in some sense related to defect-inducing early identifications. The latter, in fact, reemerged as central again and again—as did the others. And the narcissistic aspects of the rage, its emergence in response to the sense of humiliating defect, and to the puncturing of her grandiose wish to be in the center and special, were also an important part of its origins. I believe all of this is just part of the overdetermination and multiple function we regularly see in analytic work. But multiple models, I think, permit us to see them more clearly: to formulate them, remain with them, and more comfortably regard any one of them as central for a particular person at a particular time.

Or consider the learning disability, and beyond that the larger sense of defect in regard to affect control. The experience of self-as-defective had been of enormous importance to this patient, whatever the historical realities on which it was based. This experience was central to her sense of self and seems to have been developed in two directions. One is the sense of secret defect itself, an inner sense of something that ultimately defines her and that will be discovered by others. The other side is the compensatory aspect. Her great pleasure in her own humor (and her frequent use of it) is accentuated by contrast to her sense of intellectual deficit, as is an emphasis on (and the actuality of) *competence* in her whole character structure and life. The ambitious wishes to be the most important one also have a compensatory aspect. But the relation of the disability to the drive psychology is also striking: in the material given, it appears as a symbolic equivalent of castration (the "bottomless" girl) and as a *result* of the intrusion of rage on her attempts at learning (that is, as a symptom). And again it becomes central to the remembered and sought after object relationships: both in the sense of being the "unimportant" one (failure in learning, in cycling) and the "special" one (the cared-for, "defective" child).

One could say much more about these sessions. Conflict and over-determination are everywhere, as indeed they are for all significant psychological phenomena. But, I again suggest, there is no gain in trying to force these complexities into one theoretical mold. Of course one can argue that the flow of material in a clinical session does not obviate our need to formulate some more basic theory. Thus one could argue that the phenomena I have been highlighting are ultimately reducible to one or another view. But we need not take that position, and the first part of this book was an attempt to lay out an alternative view—a view of multiplicity even at the level of basic theory. Various motives are operative in each of us; various phenomena enter the clinical encounter; and they have varying centrality in different individuals. As I see it, there is more gain than loss, at present, in working with multiple models of the mind's functioning.

Each of the four clinical vignettes in this chapter was built around a session or series of sessions in which new views of the material emerged—views that can be seen as shifts in the conceptual language of understanding from drive and/or ego and/or object relations and/or self to any one or more of the others. These shifts do not go in only one direction, in my experience. No one of the domains is more basic than another. And when the shift takes place, the earlier work does not disappear from the analysis. It was not "wrong" and subsequently "correctly" understood. Rather, in cyclic and interlocking fashion each comes up again and again.

These are not typical sessions. I do not mean to suggest that these shifts come up in every session. But, in my experience, they are typical of analyses—that is, they come up in every analysis at one time or another. Ultimately they are the reflections of what we familiarly describe as overdetermination, from one perspective, or multiple function, from another. Sandler (1981), in his discussion of wished-for role relationships that can carry in them libidinal aims as well as other object-relational wishes, such as for safety, is clearly thinking along the same lines. And Jacob Jacobson (1983) also works similarly in his demonstration of drive and of "representational world" concepts in the material of particular sessions.

In my experience of my own clinical work, this way of working does not for the most part entail a self-conscious application of different conceptual languages to the clinical work. Usually I am struck by the shift, if I notice it as a shift at all, after the fact. It does not feel like a shift. It just feels like doing analysis with a patient, being alert to a wide range of phenomena and occasionally having the experience of understanding something—an experience that is conveyed to the patient in this way or that. But the *this*'s and *that*'s, upon after-the-fact examination, turn out to extend across the full array of what I have been referring to as the four psychologies of psychoanalysis.

CHAPTER 8

Summaries of Psychoanalyses

MY INTENT IN the previous chapter was to give a sense of the flow of within-session material as it is varyingly conceptualized along lines of drive, ego, object relations, and self experience. In the present chapter, by contrast, I present overviews of completed analyses. Here my aim is to give some sense of the conceptually differentiable range of contents that come up in work with individual analysands and, additionally, the varying forms of organization—the personal hierarchies—by which these are bound together. I do not mean to suggest that there are a limited number of types of such hierarchies, nor that there are "types" at all. They vary as much as individuals vary. But the concept of personal hierarchies nicely captures the very idea of that variation plus the idea that *some* inner organization of the multitudes of phenomena is present in everyone.

I shall not develop a picture of any organizational elegance within these personal hierarchies. The term is just an umbrella concept subsuming the many different kinds and degrees of organization—tight or loose, blended or sharply demarcated, coequal or hierarchical—seen among phenomena of the several psychologies in actual analyses. And of course for some (perhaps all) of the individuals to be reported on, drive, object relations, or self theorists could interpret the material entirely (or almost entirely) in their own terms. That is one of the reasons I argue for multiplicity.

A PAINFUL EXPERIENCE OF SELF IN A TIGHTLY ORGANIZED PERSONAL HIERARCHY

Mr. E, a thirty-five-year-old free-lance buyer of fine antiques for wealthy individuals, came seeking treatment when the approaching death of his father restimulated many childhood memories of a painful sort. Analysis seemed a natural route for him to follow when in distress; an older brother and two younger sisters were or had been in analysis as well. Unmarried and childless, he had nonetheless been living with a woman in a stable relationship for some ten years.

Mr. E described himself in his first session as being generally out of touch with his feelings, overcontrolled, and therefore not enjoying life to the fullest. He warned me that he was a "pleaser"; he knew how to give people what they wanted, to accommodate them, and he hoped that this would not become a danger to the treatment. He feared that I might be taken in by it, fooled into thinking he was doing better than he was. He felt compelled to be a pleaser, but he could not quite say why; he knew, though, that he wanted people to like him. He also described frequent periods in which he felt "just awful" when people didn't respond to him sufficiently. He was unable to describe this feeling in greater detail at this point. However, it rapidly became more clear and central once the treatment began—the reason being that the conditions of the analytic encounter, not seeing what response he was getting and often hearing only silence from the analyst, stimulated and highlighted his feeling "awful." He then described it as a terribly needy feeling, "the most awful feeling of my life," something that seemed like it had always been with him, something that could be satisfied only from the outside. Pleasing others was his way to woo them so that they would give him the liking and the acknowledgment that made this feeling decrease in intensity, or even temporarily reverse. After we began the treatment he described how he made inner "deals" between himself and others. He would be nice to them in such-and-such a way for such-and-such a time period, and then they would appreciate him in some way that fit the particular situation. Of course, this rarely worked out—the other person not having been party to the deal—and then Mr. E would feel angry.

One thing did become quite clear very soon after the analysis had begun. That is, in spite of his initial complaint that he felt overcontrolled and out of touch with his feelings, he was quite psychologically minded and in fact was very much in touch with his feelings—predominantly sadness and this "awful," "needy" state—though it was true that he would often squelch his feelings in the effort to please others and to accommodate them.

The patient's father had run a small retail business during all of the patient's growing up years. The memories that had been restimulated by the father's impending death—memories that had never been lost but that were now more vivid and painful affectively—had to do with his father's nonacknowlegment of him. This had two threads, each mentioned in the first consultation sessions but expanded and detailed throughout the entire course of the analysis; together they created in him (as recalled) that awful/needy feeling in his childhood, and the effort to please. One of the threads involved his experience of his father's treating him as though he did not exist—no greeting in coming home after work, no pride in any of his son's accomplishments, no interest in his interests; scores of such moments were mentioned during the analysis and, of course, readily reexperienced in the transference. The second thread was more concrete and became a leitmotif in the treatment, something we always referred back to. "Helping out" was the phrase we began to use for it. For years—from early childhood to his mid-teens—the patient was required to help out in the father's retail business on weekends. It did not matter that his friends were out playing, that he wanted to join a club, pursue a hobby. Weekend after weekend was spent helping out (and the patient often experienced the analysis this way—he was helping out; it was really for me, not for him). Worse, the patient remembered those weekends as times when he lived in dread of his father's rage. The slightest wrong move on his part would trigger that rage. If he did not respond quickly enough when his father wanted something or made a demand, rage would follow. One particularly painfully remembered period was when his father undertook to remodel his retail establishment on Sundays. For some three years the patient's Sundays were spent as a carpenter's assistant, with the whole setting producing the same fear of his father's rage, accentuated because his father now held "dangerous" tools while enraged. Altogether the experience produced in the youth bottled up rage, fear of his father's rage, and most centrally a sense of helpless humiliation—a feeling that he and his wishes simply did not exist for his father. (His father died about six months after Mr. E's analysis began.)

The patient's mother was described as an emaciated, sickly, weak woman, one who always rushed to please her husband, turning away from her son's needs in order to do so. At the outset and for a long time thereafter, she was a far more shadowy figure in the analysis than the father. Only gradually did it become clear how much he experienced her as abandoning him in favor of attending to his father, and also as relating to him primarily to satisfy her own needs when father was not around. She would also praise his accomplishments excessively and indiscriminately so that he took only a sinking sense of nonrecognition even from that praise, especially as he got older. She herself was so much oriented to pleasing others that she would say different things from moment to moment, contradicting herself in her rush to accommodate. As the analysis progressed, and as I heard about events in the life of the family, it came to seem to me that the patient, while playing out his role in the family dynamics, was nonetheless now an accurate reporter of the character and behavior of each of his parents.

I shall give just one other piece of the history before proceeding. All through his childhood the patient had what he called a nightmare. It was an image and sense of himself as growing smaller and smaller, tiny and disconnected from everyone and everything. In one frightening episode during his elementary school years, he "had the nightmare while awake," the same shrinking feeling. This occurred around the time of an episode that came to be seen as having many parallels to the nightmare. He had performed in a school play and felt very proud of himself. In school the next day, "I was very cocky." But then the teacher, seeing his cockiness (this of course is how the patient experienced it), said something that cut him down, and again he felt that small feeling—this time with humiliation. Both this episode and the nightmare came, during the subsequent analysis, to be seen (a) as reflective of the small, humiliated sense of self stemming from the history of actual intrafamilial relationships and (b) as the expression of his conviction that he had a tiny penis (compared with his father's). Fright in relation to the shrinking of the penis during detumescence was also present during his childhood. But more of that later.

I bring this patient as an example for two reasons. First, phenomena of several of the psychologies were quite prominent in the work. Sexual and aggressive urges, repetitions of old object relations via identification and/or new editions in new relationships, and a primary experience of self as belittled and unacknowledged were all actively seen and worked with during the course of the analysis. And second, the arrangements among these phenomena in his personal hierarchy were fairly tight. The particular experience of self as needy, that "most awful feeling of my life," was always central. Thus, for example, as its relation to sexuality, aggression, and defense emerged and were analyzed, these aspects did not go on to become central in his analysis, but rather seemed to drift into the background again, with the self experience reemerging centrally in ever clearer forms.

The analysis was quite successful, as measured by changes in the patient's intrapsychic and outside life. The main therapeutic direction went from his seeing the needy state as one that he passively endured at the hands of others to his seeing it as one that he now created through repetition, expectation, emotional attachment to it, and use of it for defensive purposes. With this understanding, and of course analysis of innumerable other issues in relation to it, the "awful" inner state substantially altered and the patient became able to feel much more content with his inner life and, as he periodically said, "able to feel OK even in a less than satisfying world."

In the analytic work of the first year, most of the material thus far described became known. In the sessions, a central and repetitive complaint was that I did not acknowledge him. He said that he needed me to intervene; he had "nothing to say"; I didn't let him know what I thought of him; I didn't care about him. These experiences were vivid and painful for him. Yet he could always manage to stand outside of them, at least for moments. He was in fact rarely short of "things to say," even though his experience was the opposite, and he could see that my silence sometimes led him to feel that what he had to say was not good enough. He also recalled, and often reminded me, that (as he understood it) he had seduced a prior therapist into meeting his needs, being a friend, and he made clear that he did not want that to happen again. The "danger" that he had warned me of in the first session, that his "pleasing" me would fool me into thinking he was doing fine, was now extended to the "danger" that I would try to meet his neediness by becoming his friend, something he both wanted and did not want.

I can give a sense of how some of what were to become the central issues of the analysis emerged in the first year by describing selections from a number of sessions. First, I shall sketch some of the interplay between issues of sexuality, anger, and of his painful sense of self, drawing first on two sessions (three months into the treatment). The woman that Mr. E lived with, whom I shall call Serita, often traveled in relation to her work. Mr. E resented it, believing that she could do otherwise and avoid the traveling, and of course experienced it as a nonacknowledgment of him, a failure to satisfy his neediness. She returned after one such trip and he gave her a new negligee as a gift. His inner deal was that he had pleased her, and she was now to please him by wearing it. She, on the other hand, worn out from her travels and in a low mood because her work had not gone well on the trip, wanted only to fall into bed and asleep. The patient was angry. She was a "nonentity," he said, this being his way of expressing his anger at her at this moment. As he spoke, it seemed to me that what he was saying was quite the reverse. He wanted her to do as he wished, to be his sexual object. What bothered him was that she had a will of her own, that she was (in a term I offered to him later in the session) an entity. I suggested that he was attempting to reverse the situation where he was a nonentity with his father, an object to be bent to his father's will. (I thought, at this point, that he was using sexuality as a form of anger and in order to bolster himself and reverse his sense of not mattering, of nonentity, because she had gone away.) The patient was struck by this. He immediately recalled an intense sexual relation from his adolescence. There the female was totally passive; he could do anything to her. It actually made him terribly uncomfortable. Serita was the opposite. When he met her he was attracted to her independence; at the same time he now often hated it.

A few sessions later a similar interweaving of sexual, aggressive, and self-feeling issues emerged. In this session, I was seeing the sexual and aggressive issues as primary, the needy self as a defensive cover; the patient's associations to my intervention altered this view for me. (These conceptual formulations are retrospective. At the time, I felt I was simply doing my work as an analyst.) The patient began the session by telling me that he was feeling needy—"that always comes up here"—and he was angry at Serita. They were trying to work out some plan and he felt he couldn't get heard. She wasn't responsive to him; it was as if he didn't matter. He said something about the pervasiveness of those feelings, and this somehow triggered the memory of a dream from the night before. He was in a dentist's chair; something happened and he ended up just sitting out in the rain. Then he was with an old girlfriend whom he had known since kindergarten. He was rubbing her breasts. His associations went to a wide range of sexual memories and incidents of anger. Strong feelings of both sorts were vividly expressed in the memories. I said: "You began by telling me that your 'needy self' always comes up here. Today it looks like that may be a cover story, not *the* story. It's striking how much sex and anger lie behind the cover." The patient's first association seemed confirmatory. He recalled (and told me for the first time) that he slept in his parents' bedroom until he was seven years old. (In retrospect I would say that he was "pleasing" me by giving this association to my interpretation—see the next session to be reported below.) He next went back to the needy feeling. It was like "an old friend" when he talked about it. Though painful, it was familiar. Somehow "it felt like a comfort." (He had already told me in prior sessions how much he lets himself get into experiences of sadness. Much later on he was able to describe how the sadness gave him a sense of taking care of himself, recognizing his neediness, as he wished others had done.) Then his third association (following my intervention) was another memory—of a time when his mother forgot to pick him up at school and he was left crying in the rain (as in the dream); he recalled the comforting sense of being justified in his rage at her for making him feel so unimportant as to be forgotten. I said nothing at this point, but the sense of "comfort" that appeared in his last two associations, plus the second reference to rain, gave these associations a sense of genuineness, of fit. Of course they could be seen as a move back to the comforting cover story of his needy self. And I do not doubt that some of that may have been in it. My impression of the overall analysis however, something that had to press itself upon me because it did not readily fit into my way of thinking at the time, was that the cover story (in contrast to my interpretation) indeed *was* the story, was the central affective issue and conflictual organizer of his life. (I am not trying to prove a specific case for self pathology; my main argument is in fact that multiplicities of organization are indeed universal. Other cases to be described will show different centers and different degrees of *centeredness* on that center.)

Another session two months after the previous one again demonstrated this interweaving of issues. He had been talking a great deal about sexual matters the day before. This day he came in and said that he was unsure whether all of that talk about sex was really to please me. This became the session's theme. Talk about sex might please me. But sex was a way he could feel pleased, he could feel recognized. He remembers that when he couldn't get a teen girlfriend to give him something sexually, he felt "she doesn't care about me," the start of that same needy, "unrecognized" feeling. He recalled another girlfriend "who gave me her bare breast for my birthday"; *that* made him feel acknowledged; he mattered (and recall the previous dream where rubbing an old girlfriend's bare breasts followed his being left sitting in the rain). He remembered that his former therapist had said that sex seemed to be an affirmation for him. (Some three years later the patient told me, with insight, as though he was then just seeing clearly the place in his life of something he had known about all along, that he became good at sex as an adolescent and later. He had found that that was a sure way he could get the acknowledgment he sought; he felt noticed, not needy. I'm reminded here of Fairbairn's [1941] point that the infant is object seeking but that, early on, it is only through the oral zone that he or she can seek contact and connect. Here, Mr. E tells us he could use the genital zone— sexuality—to connect in the way that he felt he needed to, which here was to feel affirmed.)

Another pair of sessions from the first year highlight the interweaving of anger and the sense of self. Mr. E came in one day on the edge of his "awful" feeling, and gradually fell more fully into it. He felt he had nothing to say, was just talking so that he wouldn't be saying absolutely nothing. But slowly over the course of the session, hints began to appear regarding an incident that angered him. However, he was not clearly aware of the anger. His communication to me was indirect, tangential. After a while I told him that I did not know what it was about but I thought I heard him alluding again and again to an incident with a relative of his that seemed obviously disturbing to him. He picked up on it easily. He had been disinvited to a particular family gathering that he had initially been invited to, and he was angry as could be. But it was only as the session came to an end that he had become aware of incipient rage in the session itself; he wanted to scream, clench his fists, pound the wall alongside the couch. "I don't know what to do with my anger; it feels like a total frustration" [because, hoping that the relative would still like him, he couldn't express it at all].

He came in the next day and his whole bearing and sense of self were altered. He was much more real sounding, with none of the needy anguish in his voice. He was fully aware of his anger and had told his relative just how he felt. In two unrelated incidents since the prior session (unrelated except that they occurred while he was in this more real sounding, less needy, state) he had been able to express his anger at Serita and at a colleague, each time in relation to injustices that he felt in relation to them. While not now angry at me, he was atypically forceful in speaking to me. He "didn't want to just make an adjustment" to his anger and put it aside, as he knew he could do. Gradually, however, in the session, he worked his way into doing just that, and his "awful" state came to the center again. I pointed out the oscillation, and he was able to recall incidents from the past in which the expression of anger was accompanied by a sense of worthwhileness, and "accommodation" by the "awfulness," in a number of situations—with relatives, Serita, and me.

It is no surprise, of course, that anger should produce a forceful inner feeling; it can be a self-defining affect if one owns it, is active in relation to it (in Rapaport's [1953] sense), and not its passive victim. But in Mr. E we later came to see not only how good he could feel about himself when he was (in his mind, justifiably) angry but also (a) his use of the familiar needy state as a *defense* against the anger (which, in circular fashion, he feared would lead to his being disliked and, hence, becoming needy) and (b) his *flight* to the needy state to hold on to the old object attachments (to father especially, but also to mother) which were bound up with that state and which were threatened by his anger.

Having introduced, in this last point, some of the links between his needy/awful state and his old object ties, I should like to give a couple of other illustrations, again from the first year, showing the intimate tie of the particular self state to his inner world of identifications and internalized object relationships.

In one session around the time just referred to, Mr. E told of an incident in which he "pleased" Serita in a phone conversation rather than express the anger that he was in fact feeling. He then managed to repeat the "pleasing" behavior in the session in relation to me. I pointed this out, and it readily triggered the old memories of pleasing his father, helping out. After a long time at this recall, he paused, and he asked himself aloud for the first time: "Where's my mother in all of this?" He went on to answer his own question:

"I always had the sense that if I didn't please my father, he'd be angry at my mother. In a way, my mother sent me to please him, to help out. I think I even felt that my mother and I were a team. She 'handled' my father in that way—or *we* did." "Pleasing" was thus his role in this particular family drama.

We garnered another perspective on this several sessions later. He was angry at Serita, and also at me, for (each in our own way) "not paying attention" to him. It was, he said, like when his mother turned her attention to his father, away from him, when father came home from work; he didn't remember being angry then, but he felt the loss of attention and felt awful. But, "So what?" he said, challenging me. "So I see this. I still have the feelings."

I said that it sounded like he was looking for a fight with me.

He responded: "I was looking for a fight with Serita when I came home last night. I expected her to be busy with her own work, to have no time for me, and I was already angry when I walked through the door."

I said: "It sounds like you are not only that 'poor little boy' looking for attention, but that you are your father—expecting it, demanding it." This interpretation produced a flood of confirmatory associations to incidents in which he was indeed just like his father in just that way.

My point in these initial remarks has been to demonstrate that the awful/needy self state that was at the center of the patient's experience was internally tied to the dynamics of sexuality, aggression, defense, identification, and internalized object relations. It was, in the first year and throughout, the center to which Mr. E kept returning. While productive analytic work was done around it in each spur into the related drive, defense, and object relational issues, it always retook center stage.

I want to bring out one more illustrative point with material from the first year. My impression rapidly came to be that the patient had indeed had a psychologically abusive experience at the hands of his father all through his childhood, producing the needy, unacknowledged experience of self. But I came to believe equally that the patient actively reproduced this experience in the present, that it had come to have many meanings and serve many functions for him. I tried to show him his active role in it; this was one of the main therapeutic thrusts of the work. Thus, in a session in our second month, when he was describing problems between himself and Serita in terms of her not being sufficiently there for him emotionally, I was able to show him how, in the particular instance, it flowed from something inside him—the deals and expectations he brought to the situation. The patient was always interested in this kind of idea when it came up, but of course generally fell back into the experience of what others *were doing to him* (actually, *not doing for him*). But the part of him that had warned me in the first consultation not to be fooled by his pleasing side, not to become his friend as a previous therapist had done, was clearly present. Thus, in a session several months into the treatment, following one where (I learned) he had felt I was being too kind, too reassuring, he came in and reported a dream. He was on a car ride with his roommate. The ride was "soft, out of touch with the bumpy ground." His associations went to the previous session. I was the roommate; last session I disappointed him. He didn't want that out-of-touch kind of analysis, that reassurance—"That's just a lot of surface shit." He wanted to get deeper into himself. Associations to parallel situations at work followed, and the session ended with his sense that he would continue to be angry at me if I let him "get by" as he always had done; he didn't want that any longer. The sense of internal responsibility for his state, and his wish to be helped to alter it from within, was clear here—and progressed over time.

The place of *inner* activity, of the role of his own wishes, was again expressed clearly by him in a session toward the end of the first year. Once again a report of being unacknowledged, needy, feeling awful—this time at a large social gathering. I was able to show him, with details of his reporting, how his attitude—"No one cares about me; I have to try to please them"—was not *responsive* to his current experience, but *imposed* upon it. He saw it readily. And he elaborated on it, adding to the meaning of the word *imposed*. Not only does he impose (that is, bring) these attitudes but he also imposes on (that is, demands attention from) others, just as his father did but as he couldn't do with his father. He asked aloud: "Why would I keep doing this?" And he answered himself: "I guess I want to see if I can make it come out differently this time. And, if I can't, at least I'll feel vindicated about what I believe about people's attitudes towards me." Here, then, the internalized object relation is seen in relation to the needy self state—but now along lines suggesting increased *ownership* of responsibility for his life. A sense of agency was developing with respect to his central and lifelong discomfort.

I will summarize the later years of this analysis, attempting to show how the various themes continued to develop. The analysis was many-sided.

While the awful/needy state of self experience was a kind of touchstone to which we regularly returned, I do not wish to give a one-sided view. I offer this patient's analysis as an illustration of a fairly tight hierarchical organization, in that so much in the spheres of drive, defense, and object relations revolved around that particular state of self experience; but it is not necessary for my purposes, nor does it even serve my purpose, to present a picture implying that everything reduces to that self state. Reductionism is not my aim; rather, my aim is a demonstration of manysidedness, of the applicability of the perspectives of many psychologies.

In a series of sessions a considerable expansion took place in our understanding of the specifically sexual aspects of the patient's feeling small (which, in terms of mood, for him meant awful/needy). He recalled once, as a boy, seeing his father's penis, which seemed huge to him, and this readily linked to his lifelong feeling that his penis was too small. A dream in which his foot was cut off "to lessen my pain" produced associations around bottled up anger when he felt unacknowledged, and he saw the holding back of that anger as "cutting off a piece of myself." But then the session shifted in direction. Further associations were to a penis being cut off and this in turn reminded him, first, of the remembered contrasting size of his and his father's penis, and then of a memory that had not been recalled before. As a young man he was having intercourse with a girlfriend in a room in his house; his father unexpectedly happened by and saw; but neither then, nor the next day, nor ever, did his father say a word about it. Here, too, the patient felt unacknowledged, cut off, not this time in his very *being* (as had been the case as a child) but in his *sexuality*, his manliness; his father would have made him feel like a man (he said) if he had acknowledged that he saw him in a sexual act. This session was followed by one in which he recalled his periodic fantasy, during sex, of watching another man having sex with the very woman he was having sex with. He was secondary during this sexual fantasy, an absence, inadequate. The fantasy, of course, reversed the situation when his father had seen him. (It was striking that, much later on when the patient brought up termination, he gave as one of the changes in himself the sense that he is "a real presence" during sex, he's really there and part of it—that is, not watching another but, in contrast, himself potent and existing). Following the recall of the memory of being seen by his father and the revelation of his fantasy of watching another man, the patient was able to work well on aspects of his sexual life. He began in the next few sessions to feel stronger, less awful, less needy—with this in turn producing a feeling of being disconnected from me (the needy state being one form of continued tie to the father), and he had a sudden worry about perhaps missing a number of sessions because of a coming holiday. As I pointed out how his sense of strength produced these feelings of loss, the patient said: "How 'awful' to feel good on my own without someone doing it for me."

A few months after the series of sessions just described, a new series of sessions shed further light on aspects of his sexuality and his sense of smallness. They began with suggestions in a dream of a "grand" part of an otherwise shabby and rotting house. My question about that grandness led to recall of times in his life when he felt "grand"— in the sense of biggest and best—but this was always followed by a sense that he was being too "cocky" and would be "cut down"—as in that memory from childhood. To avoid this, he would "pass the baton" onto others—allow them to take first place—because "in my bones, I'm unsure of myself." I pointed out the phallic allusions, that his penis would be cut down, which he readily heard in terms of his continuing sense that his penis was too small. But, in the sessions following this work, he was actually feeling good about himself, not needy or awful or small. As if he were on a roller coaster, each time this feeling came, he again lost touch with himself, feared cockiness, felt I would cut him down, and began to feel needy. He recalled thinking a childhood friend's mother had a beautiful body, but this came with another memory of his own mother's being critical of that woman, a response that again made him feel like nothing, small, humiliated for thinking the reverse of what his mother said. This was followed by other spontaneous thoughts of his in a next session: he said he had a tendency toward emaciation all his life, like his mother; did she try to make him thin and sexless, he wondered; he knew that being thin made him feel inadequate, sexless, small. In that session we were able to see how pleasing me (like "pleasing" his mother by being thin, like her) squashed his sexual self, putting him back into his needy/awful self experience. This work, and much else like it, allowed us to see that the intense and central awful sense of neediness could itself be used defensively, with his settling comfortably and familiarly into that state to resolve his conflictual experience of being too dangerously sexual and "grand." Around this time, too, work referred to in the history was accomplished, in which it seemed as though his childhood nightmare of shrinking in size had origins in his sexual anxieties around his small or shrinking penis in addition to its more familiar source in his core feeling of being obliterated, of being nothing in his father's eyes. Some time after this Mr. E brought in a dream in which a man enters a room in which he is having intercourse with Serita, and announces "screw time," upon which Serita prepares to have sex with the intruder. Mr. E's associations were blocked, aimless, though he was very disturbed by the dream. Suddenly he had the thought that the analyst was the intruder and he the woman. This opened up memories of having heard passionate sexual sounds coming from his parents' bedroom in his adolescence, and wishes "just once" to know what it was like to be penetrated like a woman. He remembered vague wishes for his father to be with him like father was with patient's mother. I said: "You wished to say to your father: 'Notice me, pay attention to me,' but also 'do it in the way that will make me feel good like you do to Mom.'" This interpretation opened up a whole series of thoughts and fantasies (not actions) regarding bisexuality.

Many of these overlapping themes of sexual envy and anxiety on the one hand and feeling small and needy on the other came together in a single session late in the analysis. Over the weekend, a friend of his had been doing some construction work and my patient joined in and lent a hand. The whole incident blended in with his helping out his father those innumerable weekends when he was reconstructing his retail store. The patient began to feel needy/awful, an absence. He was readily able to see a link to his recently having felt cocky as well; he had to pull back. But as the session went on and made clear the link between helping out the friend and helping out his father, he got angry at both. "They both acted as though they knew how to use their fucking *tools* better than I did." I responded: "They both acted as though they knew how to use their *fucking* tools better." The patient had no trouble seeing the link to his fantasies of father's superior sexual equipment and capacities; and the whole session, at first richly and convincingly evocative of his helpless "unacknowledged" relation to his father in childhood, transformed into one equally richly and convincingly evocative of his conflicts—both small and grand feelings, both envy and competition—around phallic and oedipal sexuality.

While I shall not go into it as fully, a similar interweaving of themes of anger and of the awful/needy feeling was also extensively seen. The "awful" part of the needy feeling in fact came to be seen as precisely the result of an admixture of anger that he could not express because it would interfere with the wished-for recognition and care. His passive victim stance came to be understood as justifying his rage, but also as avoiding his father's rage; "my father would kill me if I stood up to him." The patient's "pleasing" others was seen as a front for his anger—both a disguise in the eyes of the other and a defense for himself. But when he began to be able to express anger—appropriately, forcefully—it felt to him that that itself was a form of pleasing me, and it took a while before it was felt as his own, owned. Again a dream brought up much of this material vividly.

Mr. E reported a long, disturbing dream centered on his having held a tiny baby inside the palm of one hand, his dropping the baby and being unable to find him, and then thinking of committing suicide himself as the only way out of the anticipated criticism for having lost him. I will not go into his numerous associations but only mention that they seemed to me to make compellingly clear the following interpretation: that he is enraged when he is emotionally "dropped" by others, but his only response is "suicide," that is, losing a sense of any self but that small and needy one. His response, to recall such an incident from the night before, seemed confirmatory. But the next day he came in saying that my interpretation "didn't feel real in my gut." (I was quite surprised; it had seemed convincing to me and I thought he had responded well to it.) He then actively (aggressively, I would say, as though showing me all that I had missed) launched into a series of thoughts about the dream that were in essence identical to those of his *and mine* of the day before. But they were additional, and they were experienced as his own. The tiny baby was himself (he said) in his childhood nightmare. He listed new incidents (linked to the dream images) where "no one cares about me" and it makes it feel "as though life is not worth living"; "I'd as soon be dead." After a rush of such associations I pointed out how strikingly he had taken possession of his own dream; no loss of self today. He responded: he doesn't know why he sometimes loses his anger and loses himself. Today he didn't feel that way. Following, now, his *enactment* of assertion within the session, I repeated essentially the same interpretation as the day before: that is, that when he is emotionally "dropped" he "commits suicide"—loses his sense of self. Now he responded: "God, does that seem real to me!" The enactment of assertiveness in the session, in contrast to the day before—which he had come to feel as more passive, helping me out—now enabled him to experience a piece of his inner reality as *real*, not as a submission to, a pleasing of, the analyst. This kind of enactment had itself come up before (and later) and was also the subject of analytic work.

Other work in the analysis seemed nicely captured by the idea of a "false self" (Winnicott, 1960a) aspect of his needy self—this when it was used as a front for adaptation to others and as a defense against sexuality and rage. But, ironically, it simultaneously felt like his most real self. Though he always had the idea that "it used to be different"—that once long ago he felt responded to—the needy self seemed like the "real" him, and he clung to it. This led again to the position of the needy self in the retention of the old object ties and as a convoluted form of identification, as described in the work of the first year.

His small and helpless self was not absent on the day that he first mentioned the thought of termination some fourteen months before we actually terminated. He had been feeling very good about himself, both in the analysis and outside, after a series of sessions wherein some good work had been accomplished. It "gave me thoughts about ending here." But he quickly added: "I doubt that *I* can make such a decision. What would you think if I did?" As he went on, he made clear that both thinking that he "no longer needed" analysis and the act itself of making such a decision were beyond what he could do by himself. (Later, the "cocky" aspect of this also emerged.) After a few more mentions of ending—not a plan, just a passing reference—it came up in a different way in another session. Again "no one noticed" him or cared about him. But then, he said angrily: "Are you going to just let me walk out of here like that? Just because I say so? Don't you even notice me? Don't you care about me?" The termination is reexperienced as one more repetition of the early relation to father. Later he told me of "secret" gains and successes in his life—secret because they seemed uncomfortably cocky even as they seemed to justify termination. He had indeed changed in many ways and was able much more consistently to do his own analytic work in the sessions.

My intent in this summary of Mr. E's analysis is not to give a full picture of either the analytic process or its therapeutic outcome, but to demonstrate the interweaving of the phenomena of the several psychologies. So I shall end with a report of one session in which two dreams were reported; this session came soon after we had together agreed on a termination date.

The patient began: "I had a dream, or maybe it was two dreams, last night. In the first, I had been on a long trip and I was soon going to get home. I was looking forward to it. But I had met some other man on the trip, and I had really come to love him. But now it was time to say goodbye. I was on some kind of truck, and I was going to take the last leg of this journey alone. I got off the truck to hug him goodbye. He appreciated my telling him about my loving him, but he was uncomfortable with the hug. He allowed it just for a second, and then he drew back.

"In the second dream, I was on a bed. There was a couple at the edge of the bed. I'm not sure I even saw them, I have no image of them. But between them and me was another man. And he leaned over and began to suck my penis. I wasn't at all aroused. He did it for just a moment, and then he stopped.

"I guess the friend I was saying goodbye to was you—oh, where do I get off saying that! I'm prepackaging it. For all I know he was me, I was both of them. Let me see if I can just see what comes to mind.

"His discomfort with the hug reminds me of my thoughts about how I'd say goodbye after my last session here, at the end. Would I just say goodbye, or hug you, or shake your hand? I've talked about that before. I just don't know. But as I'm saying this I'm suddenly getting filled with sadness. You know, it came like a wave. It went over me, covered me, then passed. It was just for a moment. It's as though I'm uncomfortable with being enveloped by it."

At this point I said: "Perhaps you are, after all, both figures in the dream. The friend allows the hug for just a moment, but is uncomfortable with it. Just as you can only be enveloped by your sadness for a second before you get uncomfortable with it."

MR. E: "That feels right. But that sadness has always been so important to me. . . . I don't know what to say about the second dream."

ANALYST: "Before you go on, what comes to mind about the truck in the dream?"

MR. E: "Nothing, I guess. You know, that's not true. I often do that. I have an association and feel 'that doesn't count.' Always like I'm unimportant. But what I remembered was. . . ." (He went on to describe an incident from ten years earlier when he rather impetuously, but constructively from the point of view of following his own interests, drove such a truck. He also recalled that his father was connected with a trucking firm at one point in his career, and he told me the details. Then he returned to the second dream.)

"That bed that I was on had a pillow [feeling my couch pillow with his hand] like this. The man who sucked my penis had a moustache. . . . You know what came to mind when I said he had a moustache? There's an old photo of my father with a moustache when I was about four years old. After that he never had one. My mother always tells the story of when I was little, and my father had no moustache and I saw that photo, and I cried and said, 'I want the daddy with the moustache.'

"I don't know what to say about the couple. Nothing comes to mind. . . . I wasn't at all aroused by the sucking. The man doing the sucking was about thirty-five years of age, and he had fair hair, and was tall and thin. You know, he looked like me actually. That's odd."

ANALYST: "That has a certain symmetry, doesn't it? In the first dream you turn out to be both characters—the one saying goodby and the one uncomfortable with being enveloped. And here again you have the thought that you're both the man sucking and the man being sucked. Somehow that holds together."

MR. E: "You know what I remembered when you said that? It's like things fit together perfectly. I was reading an essay in a magazine by some psychologist over the weekend and he talked about therapy as a perfect melding together of the patient and therapist. It really touched me. That's what I feel I've had here. Like a perfect fit."

Nearing the end of the hour, I said: "There are three important men in your life—your father, me, and you—and we all keep coming up in the dreams. I think the dreams express your loving feelings toward me, the wish to hug me, the feeling that I've taken perfect care of you. But I think they also express the wish that you had had that experience with your father— that you *both* were involved with trucking, that he took care of you, somehow nonarousingly, by sucking your penis, that you could have 'the daddy with the moustache.' And yet, I think the dreams also express your feeling that now you'll have to be taking care of yourself—sucking your own penis, feeling the waves of sadness."

Mr. E responded with a wistful half-laugh: "I guess so. That seems to be how it is. [But then more forcefully:] You know, that's what that essay was about too. About how that perfect blending is to allow the patient to understand himself, and then to use it or not as he wishes. But for himself. Not for his therapist, not for any theory, but for himself. That's always been what it's been like here. My doing for myself."

He lapsed into silence and, after a minute or so, I ended the session. I was struck, here close to termination, by the patient's capacity to work on his own. But, from the point of view of my present purpose, equally striking is the weaving together of issues of sexuality and of self worth—the wish to be attended to expressed in the language of sexuality (sucking his penis), and his capacity for self care similarly.

In summary, I have attempted to give a small but representative sample of Mr. E's analysis. It was many-sided but the needy/awful experience of self— one that rapidly became clear at the outset as his central affectively painful experience—retained centrality throughout. It seemed to have its origins in the repeated relation to his father throughout childhood, an external experience, but it was certainly worked over in innumerable ways internally and achieved multiple meanings and functions in relation to conflict over sexual and aggressive urges and in relation to internalized object relations, later actively reproduced in his life by the patient. I did not particularly expect that the analysis would follow this path; if anything, I expected that the early childhood experience with father would lessen in centrality as other intrapsychic transformations took over. But that was not the way the analysis went. Following the patient, I found we kept coming back to that painful experience of self in relation to father (primarily; mother, secondarily), though I also found we moved down intrapsychic paths that seemed to be thoroughly like what I have come to know analyses are like. The work went on in the languages of drive and defense, of self experience and the adaptations it wrought, and of early object relations and identifications repeated ad infinitum. But, it now seems to me, this is the stuff—in varying shapes and with differing emphases—of all analyses.

OEDIPAL CENTRALITY IN A MODERATELY
LOOSE HIERARCHY

Mr. F was forty-two years of age when he sought analysis because of problems he was encountering at work. He was an attorney, specializing in labor arbitration, and the problems were of two sorts: first, he found himself to be competitive with his colleagues in ways that seemed to him inappropriate and excessive, and he was troubled by it; and second, and even more troubling, he felt he was managing to undo himself in his work, to perform far less well than he might. This latter was very familiar to him; though he had at times shown real excellence in various areas, an excellence that had often been recognized by others as well, more often he performed at a mediocre level, and followed specific successes with dramatic declines.

Mr. F had many interests. He loved cooking in his spare time, and had taken courses in culinary arts; he was an avid birdwatcher; and he sang in a men's chorus, at times singing solo baritone parts. He was quite aware of the image of attorneys as "hard-boiled and competitive" (as he saw it), and took pleasure in the contrast between his interests and that image. In fact, he was proud of his work in labor arbitration, seeing that as a peacemaking activity. That intensified his distress at his competitiveness, something that had surfaced many times in his life and that he tried to keep in check. Mr. F had had many relationships with women but had never married.

He was the firstborn and only son in a family of three children. His father had also had ambitions to be an attorney, but he had married young and had soon had to support a growing family, which led him to give up that dream. He turned his back fully on further schooling in his disappointment, and got into a business where he eventually became quite successful. But his personality had changed with this change in life course. He became morose, isolated, and disinterested. While his son wished to think the best of him and actively to hold on to his love for his father (for reasons that will become clear in a moment), the analysis rapidly brought to the fore the patient's deep and continuing sense of the father's emotional unavailability. The father, incidentally, had also loved singing, but informally, of the singing-in-the-shower variety. That, too, he gave up when he gave up his educational dreams. The patient's mother was recalled as emotionally volatile, quick to a frightening degree of anger that, to make matters worse, seemed unpredictable and irrational to Mr. F as a child. The parents fought frequently, but the marriage had nonetheless been stable.

When Mr. F was just under eighteen years of age his father died. Though the death had been expected, it nonetheless came as a sudden shock to Mr. F. The circumstances were these: Mr. F had done very well in high school (his tendencies to follow success with failure had not yet begun), and he entered a college away from home just after his sixteenth birthday. Soon thereafter, it was discovered that his father had lung cancer; the family, including the patient, understood that his death was coming. During the period following the diagnosis, however, the patient developed a much warmer relationship with his father; it was extremely important to him, following, as it did, years and years in which he felt deeply the sense of his father's isolation and distance. They had frequent phone conversations that were satisfying to the patient and spent much time doing things together at home during school vacations. The actual death came more rapidly than expected in the final period. It was just before the patient's final examinations of his second year; and his mother, rationalizing that the death was expected and not wanting to disrupt her son's exams, chose not to inform him. Thus it was that Mr. F learned of the death only about a week later, upon his return home; he recalls being hit by the news as though it were "a blow to my chest." It was later learned, during the analysis, that his reaction to the death began to be suppressed and denied after that initial strong reaction. He entered therapy soon after that for about a year, at college, around "problems with relationships." When I first met Mr. F, the effort to hold on to a loving view of his father was holding its own against awareness, simultaneously present, of father's lifelong emotional distance.

As subsequently revealed in the analysis, the death interacted with developmental events in Mr. F's late adolescence that led to further emotional complications for him. When he had first reached his teens, he began to enjoy the idolizing relationship that his two younger sisters had with him. But he was also aware of the thought that he was a better father to them than his father was to him. And then, in the period after the father's death, especially on holidays at home, when his mother turned in many ways to lean on her almost grown son, he was also aware of feeling like "the man of the house," a better husband to his mother than his father had been. In this context, the father's death provoked powerful feelings of loss—accessible from very early on in the analysis—but also of guilt and rivalry, accessible only more slowly.

The patient recalled his childhood self as sickly, weak, and fearful. He was full of aches and pains and worried about his body. He felt strong feelings of being "defective," feelings that he attached to particular (minor) bodily abnormalities. This sense of self radically contrasted with his "man of the house" sense of power, and the two contrasting states became central in the analysis in innumerable ways.

Issues related to drive, ego, internalized object relations, and self experience all appeared in Mr. F's analysis in varying forms. To the degree that there was a central organizing thread, here it was the oedipal constellation, broadly conceived, and it involved the compound of wishes and relationships in respect to both father and mother, varyingly with sexual, aggressive, and rivalrous components, and linked to the psychological issues of various stages of Mr. F's life. But this "central thread" was not quite as central as the thread of the needy/awful state in Mr. E. There, each analytic foray into other domains seemed to end up circling back to that central state. In Mr. F, while everything is of course interconnected as it is in anyone, in retrospect it seems to me that we often were working in the conceptual domain of any one or more of the several psychologies without necessarily touching back on that central thread. Descriptively, the organization of the personal hierarchy here was less tight.

My aim in what follows is, once again, only to indicate some of the work within the domains of each of the psychologies. And again, this is, of course, a conceptual abstraction from a continuous process. I shall describe some phenomena with respect to the repetition of old internalized object relations, then some aspects of ego function, then the sexual conflicts of the oedipal constellation, and finally, in looking at a particular experience of self in Mr. F, I shall follow interwoven threads into each of the four psychologies.

The death of Mr. F's father rapidly became central in the analysis—first in terms of memories of his initial painful response to the loss, but simultaneously in terms of the freeing up of his blocked mourning. After the diagnosis of the father's cancer, their new and warmer relationship had become immensely important to Mr. F. On holidays, his father would spend time with him, going places around the city; and their conversations would include (as the patient recalled them) various kinds of advice on life and on growing up. One of the patient's responses to the death was a painful, lost feeling that he described frequently early in the analysis. In fact, in wandering around the city without his father (after the death) he had gotten momentarily lost on two occasions, enacting his internal state. We later came to understand many things about the "lost" feeling. It harked back to his lonely, sickly, fearful experience of himself as a young child, with the sense that he was at risk for falling back into that state. But it also served to help hold on to a treasured image of father as concerned guide, and thus served to ward off his anger at father's earlier lifelong emotional unavailability. And further, it held on to the father as a wished-for presence, this in the face of the anxiety over his oedipal fulfillment as the "man of the house"—more dangerous after father's death. But all of this emerged later, and slowly. The first entry of the feeling of being lost into the analysis was in a form that sought the repetition of that lost relationship but served as a resistance in the transference. He would give associations haltingly, unsure how to proceed, and always waiting for a cue from me. After a while, when it became clear that he was aware of doing that, I said, "I guess if you follow your own thoughts you may get lost again"; the patient, profoundly moved, saw readily how he was behaving so as to attempt to reproduce the (traumatically lost and intrapsychically required) object relationship.

Not long after this a much more magnified expression of the same phenomenon became clear. We had been speaking of his experience of himself as my "loyal son"; his inner idea (which now became explicit) was that as long as he worked hard as my loyal son in the treatment I would rescue him; I would preserve him from feeling lost. He began to become aware that he brought in problems in order to be "found" (that is, understood). It didn't much matter what I said or what he learned; he just wanted to come away with the feeling of having been found. In fact, he noticed that he sometimes made his life experiences more confusing than they were in actuality, so that the experience of being found, understood, would be more satisfying. Thus, the whole intent of his approach to treatment was to achieve a repetition of a lost relationship, to act out within the treatment, rather than to get on with his life. As soon as this was put into words, he realized that a previous therapy that he had had was entirely experienced that way. Each session would see his coming in in a state of confusion only to be "guided" back to steady ground.

But it was not only the more satisfying relationship to the father that was re-created through repetition. To give but one example that later became significant in the work: Mr. F had a long and problematic relationship with a woman (whom I shall call Maria) during the first couple of years of the analysis. His anxieties and inhibitions in regard to their sexual closeness were one of the major routes into his oedipal attachments and fantasies. Maria's chronic unreliability and her emotional distance took a long time to become clear because so much of the relationship looked (from the standpoint of the analytic work) to be a product of his anxiety and withdrawal. Her distance well served his anxiety about closeness, in light of the oedipal significance for him of the sexual encounter. But when the problems from her side of the relationship became compellingly clear, Mr. F still had significant difficulty in detaching himself. The relationship was on-again, off-again, with the patient continually reinvesting in it long after it seemed essentially over. Only much later in the analysis, when we saw how the attachment to this unreliably available woman permitted him to hold on to the relationship to the emotionally unavailable father-of-childhood, was he able decisively to give up the relation to her. It emerged in a session in which his feelings of loss regarding his father and his fears of mourning were again ascendant. He said that he had not wanted to need any woman since he broke up with Maria, and this recalled parallel feelings of not wanting to need anyone again after his father's death. This rapidly moved into our both seeing how Maria connected him to his father. His sense of her *absence* was in fact the form of father's *presence*. No sooner was this put into words by me than the patient felt it vividly, the experience from the past being essentially identical. The powerful motive toward repetition could be revised after that insight.

Repetitions of earlier relationships, satisfying and painful, were central to the analytic work again and again. These repeated relationships had, over time as in the earlier examples, come to serve functions in relation to sexual and aggressive wishes and defense against them. But they had (and, I maintain, have for us all) a motive power in their own right (see chapter 5), and analytic work in relation to them was a significant part of the analytic process.

All core ego functions were intact in this essentially high functioning man. Aspects of ego function found their main place in the analysis (aside from his good reporting and self-observational capacities) in relation to the analysis of defense, which is interwoven in everything else I shall present. But I want to mention two of the points at which the analysis of the defense itself was highly productive, not only in freeing our access to other material but in terms of what the defense itself contained and its overall significance in the work.

The first instance I shall describe is of interest because it illustrates the warding off not of specific content, but of a whole domain of ego function—here, the experiencing of emotions. The understanding of this came in three steps and, gradually, had the consequence that the patient could allow emotions to come forth. He felt deeply, passionately, in relation to many things; the power of feelings was itself a basis for his warding them off, underlying his initial effort to present himself as thoroughly "rational"—that is, in control, not having needs, and having only well-tamed emotions. The understanding unfolded as follows. In one early session, Mr. F started the session by saying he had felt fearful "of what would happen" that day. His associations went to various feelings (not here felt strongly) which would make him feel out of control, flooded. He went on to say how feelings somehow felt like something outside of himself, or outside of the self that he felt comfortable with. They hit him as though they had an impact from the *outside*. His thoughts then went to his father—and to the news of his death, and the impact "from the outside" that that news had had on the patient. We were able to see clearly the link of internal emotions and external facts—two painful, "outside," dangerous, out-of-control things. Shortly thereafter, the patient returned to this material, but something new was now added. He spoke of his fear of feeling. "I'm afraid my feelings will be too much for me. They'll devastate me. I won't survive." Some things that he said following this remark made me wonder, and then comment, "It sounds like you feel feelings will *cause* harm." This immediately triggered a memory of the period just before his father's cancer diagnosis when the patient had been angry at him, and the first emergence of his idea that his anger had ultimately killed his father. This had been an ongoing unconscious fantasy; its beginning emergence in this session was but the start of what became a major flowering in the analysis; the fantasy and its impact extended into many corners of his intrapsychic life, but I shall not go into all of that here. Instead I want to return to the continuing work on his defense against *all* feelings. His opening statement in the session: "Feelings will devastate me; I won't survive," is the reflection of the other fantasy: "My father did not survive my feelings." A few sessions later a third aspect of the defense against feelings in their entirety emerged. He had often spoken of his fear of being "flooded" by feelings. In this session he spoke of some (to me) relatively minor feelings of annoyance and guilt in relation to a colleague at work. But *he* was quite distressed at these feelings—again fearing that they would get out of control. I asked whether there ever was a time when he couldn't control his feelings. His response: "No. Not that I recall." But then immediately, for the first time in the analysis, he recalled how he had wet the bed until he was in his early teens. He "couldn't control that," and it embarrassed him enormously. I said: "So your feelings will come in another flood." His response: "Yes. It does feel like it would be wetting the bed."

In retrospect, I see these small but significant bits of analytic work as the core of our work on this particular aspect of ego function—a defense that segregated off a whole other ego function: affects and their signal value. Emotions were as dangerous as outside news, out of control; and they could cause harm, one "would not survive them"; and he, in particular, "knows" he would lose control of them because being "flooded" was a significant part of his experience. Other things came later: memories of "out-of-control" moments, feared identification with his "out-of-control" mother. But the work just summarized was the turning point in the freeing of the patient to experience his emotions and make them part of the analysis. That this relatively small piece of work could be so effective was testament to Mr. F's active emotional responsivity all along, but a responsivity that he struggled to suppress in his effort to be "rational."

One other specific bit of ego analysis was an early turning point in the work. At about the time of his father's death, a number of additional events in the patient's life (not reported here) had also occurred, adding to the overwhelming traumatic intensity of that period. The patient told and re-told those events. He referred to it as "my story." I listened, convinced of and respecting their traumatic intensity, and allowing the patient to be heard. At times I made some contribution in relation to it—perhaps interpretive, perhaps merely giving recognition to the traumatic intensity of the events. A turnaround began when the patient came in one day saying that "I have no 'story' for today, and I'm afraid of what might come out instead." The role of the traumatic "story" as defense was now introduced. Over time we came to see how he used it as a defense against spontaneous (and conflictful) associations to sexual and aggressive thoughts. We also came to see it as a central part of his self-definition, linked to his earlier experience of himself as weak and sickly and defending against his more dangerous self experience as the competitively successful "man of the house." And finally we came to understand it as yet another form of attachment to his father; were he to move beyond the trauma and the frozen mourning it embodied he would leave his father behind, both dead and bypassed. The trauma or "story" carried his whole life history: an overwhelming event that could not be mastered, a defense against drives, a form of self-definition and maintenance of old object attachments. While the trauma *was* a trauma, it also came to accumulate other functions. Analysis of those functions contributed to the patient's ability to master the trauma, now seen in terms of its present functions as well.

I shall turn now to another small sample of the analytic work, this time on sexuality and rivalry in their oedipal constellation. In this patient, the oedipal issues were clearly most central dynamically. They were dominant in the personal hierarchy in terms of significance—as self experience issues were for Mr. E—though (as noted) the oedipal issues did not touch all *other* issues, in the way that the self experience issues did for Mr. E.

The patient initially portrayed his mother as an irrationally angry, volatile woman who aroused fear and caution in her son. For the first six months or so of the analysis, that presentation remained relatively fixed in its one-dimensional form. The first indication of change came when, after many sessions of freed-up mourning and crying over the death of his father, Mr. F came in one day and became aware of a feeling that "my mourning is passing"—this immediately followed by the ego-alien (that is, intrusive and ununderstood) thought that now he'd begin to get into things about his mother. He became anxious with this thought. Nonetheless, not much by way of associations and memories regarding mother (except regarding her feared volatile side) was forthcoming for about another three months. At that time, when the patient had turned more to his sexual experiences—and particularly to gratifying ones—he came in one day "feeling good" and proceeded to talk about several relationships with women in which he felt sexually successful and attractive. Immediately he began feeling "embarrassed" in telling me this, and he attributed it to "rejecting you as I get healthier." This rang false to me and I asked him what came to mind about the embarrassment. He said he had always felt embarrassed about being sexual—especially in front of his mother. As an adolescent, he had never wanted her to see the girls he dated or even to know that he had dates. Then he recalled another incident. He had been singing in a chorus in high school. His mother came to hear him. He felt terribly embarrassed. Certain things (he said) he associated with his father—like being attractive to women and singing—even though his father had given up singing at the time he gave up his legal ambitions and became more withdrawn. These things felt like his father's territory; he had been embarrassed to have his mother see him engaged in them.

Once the ice had been broken and the theme opened up, other associations followed rapidly in the subsequent sessions. He recalled his earlier closeness to mother as her special helper, her only son. These memories led to a rich opening into his earlier years, including his position as the non-sexual "friend" of his mother. Then came the memory of certain obsessional thoughts from childhood that seemed derivative of primal scene experiences and the efforts to deny (doubt) what was seen and heard. This series of sessions came to a close with the embarrassment theme and the theme of self as "knowing" (about sex, about primal scene) coming together in one session: the patient was talking about the many things he kept secret from his mother in his adolescence (though he made no mention of sex); he was also speaking of his many inhibitions at that time. I suggested that both the secrecy and the inhibitions reflected the embarrassment he would have felt were his mother to know he was no longer nonsexual, and that these sexual feelings were all occurring in her presence while he was at home. Mr. F responded by recalling that he is often inhibited sexually with women until the point when it is clear to both of them that they are going to have a sexual relation. It is as though (he said) once she *knows*, she's not his mother. I suggested that secrecy, then, *is* his sexual/nonsexual tie to his mother: a knower is a not-mother; a mother is a not-knower.

This work was accomplished just before the first summer's break and did not get picked up again for some time. When it did come back into the sessions it was in this way: for several sessions the patient had expressed "confusion" about "weird" thoughts that flickered at the edge of his awareness. They involved fleeting images of his mother as he masturbated, an image of himself "cut in half," and thoughts about being better than his father. Then he came in to a next session and said: "I've been straightening up everything in my house. Making it neat. I knew just what I was doing, but I felt compelled to do it. I was fleeing from my thoughts, so I wouldn't have those thoughts I was having lately." I asked what came to mind about that particular way of fleeing his thoughts. His immediate response: "That's what I was like when I was younger, when I was my mother's good [nonsexual] boy. I always kept my room neat. She praised me for it. I felt I was good." So the compulsive neatness as a defense carried out the old nonsexual object tie. While the patient felt comfortable in this session, it was followed by sessions with considerable anxiety, including recall of the earlier "nonsexual" closeness wherein he also thought his mother was "so pretty" and he loved being close to her and having physical contact.

I shall mention briefly three other threads that tied into the oedipal constellation and then summarize a pair of sessions late in the analysis where many of them came together vividly. (1) Competition with his father emerged forcefully via transference manifestations. Thus he came in one day telling how enormously he enjoyed the play *Equus*, only to realize anxiously that the putting down of the psychiatrist in that play gave him a feeling of victory over me. When he arrived early the next day and I was not yet at my office he felt smug, superior to me, but then began to worry that something had happened, that I might have gotten killed or something. This led back to his father's cancer diagnosis after the patient had been angry at him. (2) Bodily anxieties and castration imagery had come up frequently. These images stuck in his mind like the obsessional thoughts of childhood. Linked to this material, his being "good" as a child and at present (through his "good" legal work and his "good" interests: cooking, singing, birdwatching) came up. We eventually understood it as his magical incantation—his way of assuring that no harm would come to him; "If I'm good, no one will hurt me." And later, "If I'm good, I won't die" (like father). But then Mr. F became aware of his being good as itself a form of competitiveness; he was better than others and wooed his mother in this way. (3) His singing moved into center stage. An image of a blowtorch while a woman was performing fellatio on him opened up associations to penile attack—aggressively and sexually—like a urinary stream (enuresis), and in turn to his singing. He became aware of his pleasure in the "intense tone" that "flows" from his throat—for him another penetrating phallus.

As I have already said, oedipal themes were central in the analysis, and work on them led to a freeing up of the patient's functioning in his work (an initial presenting problem), to a reduction in that part of his competitiveness that he had felt troubled by (the other presenting problem), and to easier relationships with women and with his mother. The changes were progressive over time, and there was no single period when the work got done primarily or dramatically. But a pair of sessions late in the analysis illustrated the coming together of the many issues.

He came in with a dream of "warlike" images. He contrasted this to his life in which he felt things were now going so well. It was like "getting away with murder" to do so well, since all around him he saw others not doing as well. But something odd was happening recently. He kept losing his pens— first one, then another. They reminded him of the weapons in his dream.

The interpretation went in the direction of the equivalence: pen = penis = weapon, and his self-castration (losing the pens) as punishment for his competitive success, especially in light of the death of his father at just the time when the patient was turning into a man. He returned the next session aware of having had many other images of bodily damage—such as the loss of his arms—since the prior session; he was not anxious about this now. He felt he saw what was happening. But he then, with insight, told me his "real crime." He had been singing with a woman friend. He knew that, by singing well, he was actually getting her interested in him sexually, and he wanted to attract her. He knew it, and he permitted it, and he succeeded. "That was really getting away with murder." Both insight and intrapsychic freedom were increasing.

I should like to summarize one other aspect of the analytic work with Mr. F by way of illustrating the way a particular phenomenon of self-experience branched out and accumulated multiple meanings, understandable in terms of each of the four psychologies. The phenomenon appeared first in Mr. F's recall of his sense of himself as small, weak, and sickly as a young child. This was a core self-defining experience, painful to him, and marking one aspect of his continuing relation to the world—at risk, failing, frail. (After a while the patient also became aware of an internal contradiction—that he actually also felt a strong sense of himself, something which had always emanated from him, right from the moment of my first meeting with him.) As a child he felt like a "victim of crosscurrents, wishy-washy, like a marshmallow floating in the sea." There were somatic aspects too: aches and pains, a sense that minor blemishes were evidence of something wrong with his body, and picking at his body in various ways. Late in the analysis, these phenomena appeared at a much higher level, with his sense of "loss of integrity," of "deformation" of himself. But now, still early in the analysis (and continuing for some time), he told me of how he looked in the mirror when distressed; only later did I learn that this meant *very* distressed—feeling "disorganized" or "disoriented." At such times, his reflection in the mirror "soothed" him, made him "feel less fuzzy," "aware that I had borders." In spite of the serious-sounding ring of some of these reports, I never had the sense that his pathology was very primitive; and the subsequent course of the analysis confirmed that. But he certainly did at times suffer severe anxiety, which felt disorganizing to him. I will not describe our work on those issues sequentially, but instead in terms of the several directions in which it went in overlapping and cyclic ways.

One direction was toward vivid recall and some reconstruction of his very early childhood subjective state when he did feel buffeted by the crosscurrents of his mother's rages and his father's unresponsiveness. Coupled with his mother's apparently depressed, distracted, and overwhelmed state at the birth of each of his younger sisters, the patient felt either abandoned or terrified of being the object of her unpredictable outbursts of rage. This core experience of self became familiar and itself achieved motivational force as it came to embody his wish for care and his self-definition as "good," neither competitive nor dangerous. It was a state to which he could comfortably and uncomfortably return; that is, though it was a state of generally negative affective tone, it was familiar, and therefore safe. He felt he was defective, ultimately identified with his out-of-control mother. "I felt she didn't make me right; it was her fault; I was like her." As illnesses, injuries, and minor surgery occurred in his growing up years, they not only added to his sense of being defective, but they were interpreted by him in terms of that preexisting sense of self; they were proofs, evidences of his defectiveness. Castration derivatives—broken bones, enuresis—were also proof that "she didn't make me right; I was like her."

But this negative experience of self, through which he patterned, organized, and "explained" many of his experiences, was also overdetermined and multiply functional. His own anger was central to it. Early on in the analysis it became clear that denied and avoided rage touched off his experience of disorientation and his picking at his body. The picking was itself aggressive, turned on himself, and it was a masturbation equivalent; masturbation occurring in those same states would include self-soothing aspects and aggression-controlling aspects both in the accompanying fantasies and in the masturbatory actions themselves. His immediate reaction to his anger was, "I want to be rational; I want it to go away." As the work went on we were able to see one direction in which this went: toward further proof of his being rageful like mother, and therefore out of control from within as well as in the world outside. And we saw a second direction in which it went: toward character development, being "good," "above reproach," and tormented by conscience. He saw its links to the direction of his legal career. Arbitration was peace making; it would please people; and his other interests (in his mind's eye) were those for gentle and loving people.

While we saw early on that the sense of disorganization (within) or disorientation (in the world) came when he sensed his rage building, much later we saw the other side of the pincer in which the patient was trapped. When he was "too good," when he "went along" with others and accommodated, he felt a "loss of integrity." Though the characterologically tamed anger which led to his "going along" was often something he was not aware of, the anger experienced as resulting from the going along became more and more disturbing to him. If he was angry, he tried to be good; if he was too good, he became angry. And the "loss of integrity" by accommodating came to feel like a loss of bodily integrity too—a reminder of his old, familiar, sickly/weak self, and castrated. So anger or inhibition of anger took him to the same end point.

A dream of "a self-deforming sneaker" that (in the dream) he had invented, which changed shape as you stepped on something, so that it "wouldn't even crush a cockroach," led to a series of associations over a number of sessions which again highlighted the links of active aggression, defensive characterological style, and his experience of self. By this point in the analysis, he readily saw that he was the self-deforming "sneaker," both accommodating (self-deforming) and sneaky in what he accomplished with it. "I can use it to get what I want; I'm good at it; I get my way." And he could use it in analysis, "to fool you" (as resistance); "you won't know where I'm really at." But it adds to his feeling of formlessness. "I'm just a miserable chameleon." So we saw that if he got angry, he felt disorganized; but if he avoided anger by "self-deformation," "going along," he also felt "formless." Again he was caught in a pincer of his own making, the neurotic solution ensuring the continued repetition of the failed outcome. The series of sessions in which this work went on was immediately followed by the opening up of a whole new area of childhood memories—now of his fear of ever feeling angry at his father, the father having "dangerous tools" (in his workbench in their basement) which could be used as weapons.

Closely linked to all of this was the use of his incipient fear that he might "fall apart" as a means to the continuation of the relationship to the love objects of his childhood. In the transference and throughout his history, it represented a demand to be taken care of better than he felt he had been in actuality. Thus, it was a form of wished-for relationship. But it took on a new object-relational component after the death of his father. In relation to that, the picking at his body came to carry meanings of identification and rescue.

He would feel a "violence in my chest" (the site of the father's cancer), and he would tormentedly feel like picking at it to get it out.

I shall mention one last area of work in relation to these self states—here their defensive function (within the domain of the psychology of the ego). After his father's death, Mr. F went to see a therapist for about a year. How much was contributed by the therapist's intrusiveness, and how much by the patient's need to turn inward and protect himself at that period, is not clearly known; but the patient's experience was clear. He felt intruded upon, invaded, and the experience of breakdown of defensive barriers produced that same sense of disorganization. And when he "appeased" the former therapist by revealing things about himself, this also produced the "deformation," the "loss of integrity" that could only much later be described in those terms. Needless to say, the analytic process itself was feared, and readily reexperienced, as a renewal of this "invasion"—but, at this point in his life, the patient (on the evidence of the successful analysis) could clearly work with this very fear analytically. (And I shall mention one last inversion: we came to see the patient's experience of being invaded from the outside as itself also a defense against his experience of the invasion from the inside—by his own urges, feelings, and fantasies. We came to understand his numerous childhood fears in these terms—as displacements outward of these sources of danger.)

When I contacted Mr. F for his permission to publish this material, and after he had had a chance to read it, he told me something further about the end of the analysis and its subsequent effect. He recalled how he had wished never to need anyone again after his father's death. But he had come to acknowledge needing me, while at the same time he could leave me (terminate) and get on with his life. This felt like an important achievement to him. It permitted him to feel that need with a woman as well, and he had been able to marry a couple of years after the analysis ended.

I have not attempted to give a full description of this analysis, but just enough to give a sense of its manysidedness. We terminated it by mutual consent and both, I believe, felt it to have been a successful and worthwhile experience. I give it here as just an ordinary analysis—special to the participants, but in its form and content not unusual. This manysidedness—the interplay of issues of drive, ego, object relations, and self experience—is what any analysis is made up of. We may formulate our theories, or summarize our clinical work, in one or another theoretical language, but we also need not. I prefer not. And I prefer the multimodel approach right now because (a) I see no gain, and indeed potential arbitrariness, in forcing the phenomena of analysis into narrower theoretical molds and (b) because the different weighting—the differing personal hierarchies—in Mr. F leaning toward oedipal issues, in Mr. E more tightly organized around self experience—are potentially better captured in a multimodel view.

A HIERARCHY OF SELF AND OBJECT ISSUES
"UNDER" DRIVE-DEFENSE ISSUES

I shall present material on one more patient to illustrate a third personal hierarchy reflected in the unfolding of material of the four psychologies in the analysis. In this instance, however, I am able to give only a brief summary of the actual analytic material.

Mr. G, age twenty-seven, showed a subtle deadness at times in sessions, of a kind that it took me a long time to capture and put into words for him. Once I did, the patient began to notice it, recognized it as long familiar, and referred to it as "going flat" (the patient was also impotent). Aside from the metaphorical link to the impotence, gradually I came to see this as a defense which set in when threatening sexual fantasies arose. Interpretation of this defensive aspect of going flat regularly led to recall of more animated states, generally involving sexual, aggressive, or independent strivings, as well as to recall of significant aspects of the life history. This work, over the first three years of the analysis, and which I conceptualize in terms of the drive and ego (defense) psychologies, produced impressive gains in the patient's functioning: an end of the impotence and a general increase in feelings of well-being.

But then the patient's thoughts about an impending end to the analysis (which I had not suggested) produced a massive regressive return to the going flat state. The sense of deadness and obliteration of self became more pervasive than ever. This came about through an infatuation, homosexually tinged but not acted upon, with a somewhat older, powerful, and rather abusive superior at his job. He was drawn to this man and did not at first comprehend why he should be so flooded with fantasies about him; the gains he had made earlier in the analysis dropped away rapidly and a pervasive deadness, far beyond the earlier bouts of it, set in. Over a period of about a year, tormented by his fantasies about his man, he gradually recalled sexual abuse at the hands of an older brother, probably dating back to at least the patient's third year. This led to our seeing his going flat, his deadness, as a *primary* self-feeling, related to being treated like an object without will. He experienced recall of a hopeless giving in to the brother's abuse as a child, in fact going flat as he passively, hopelessly, lay on his back on the floor—overwhelmed by the brother's threats and his own flood of emotions. The absence of will and the sense of being an object was central to these experiences.

In the analysis, the core self-feeling of deadness was paralleled by his fantasized reenactments of the old internalized object relationship with the brother. I would formulate the hierarchy here as involving self and object relations issues lying "under" drive-defense issues, both sets organized in relation to the "going flat" experience.

Eventually, after almost a year of work, the infatuation with his boss was given up and the patient began to move back and forth, now more insightfully, between the issues of both phases of the analysis as we moved slowly toward a termination of the work.

My intent with the two full analyses summarized in this chapter has been to give a close-up picture of the work in order to illustrate how phenomena of each of the four psychologies find their place. Additionally, I have commented (for each of those patients, and a third) on aspects of the organization of the several sets of phenomena—the personal hierarchies in which we find them. Though I cannot assume that all readers will be convinced of the clinical and conceptual utility of thinking in terms of the phenomena of the four psychologies, I hope that the material presented in this and the preceding chapter has at least made clear my points of reference for the theoretical arguments advanced earlier in this book.

PART III

APPLIED

Ɪɴ THIS SECTION, I use the concepts outlined in part I as the basis for a discussion of a number of issues in psychoanalytic developmental and clinical theory. In that sense it is an applied section—an application of the presented ideas to other questions in psychoanalytic theory. It is not applied psychoanalysis in the usual sense—say, applications to literature or anthropology—that is, to issues outside of psychoanalysis proper. The four chapters to follow address the following areas: the concept of preoedipal pathology; the concept of ego defect; the nature of developmental phases, particularly in light of the critique of the symbiotic phase from e standpoint of the new infancy research; and the mutative factors in psychoanalysis and psychoanalytic psychotherapy. Each discussion takes off from a four psychologies point of view.

CHAPTER 9

The Concept of Preoedipal Pathology

IN HIS BOOK *The Basic Fault*, Michael Balint (1968) wrote:

> It often happens in a science that an unhappy choice of name leads to
> misunderstandings, or prejudices the unbiased study of the problem. In
> order to avoid these risks the two mental levels [that he has been dis-
> cussing] should be called by terms that are independent of each other.
> Just as the Oedipal level possesses its own name derived from one of its
> main characteristics, so the other level should have its own, and should
> not be called pre-something else—certainly not pre-Oedipal, because
> it may coexist with the Oedipal level, at any rate as far as our clinical
> experiences go. (p. 16)

Balint used this argument as part of his introduction to what he called the
area of the basic fault. It serves as an introduction for my purposes as well.

The concept of preoedipal pathology is in danger of becoming a wastebasket term, linking many things together that would better be differentiated from one another. In defining certain forms of pathology as "preoedipal," we are saying more about what they are *not* (that is, that they are not oedipal, or not originally or primarily oedipal) than about what they *are*. It is like dividing the world into analysts and nonanalysts or schizophrenics and nonschizophrenics. The classification is useful for some purposes, but surely the "non" group can be better described and internally differentiated than these classifications suggest. The concept preoedipal purports to say *something* about those other regions of pathology—that is, that their sources lie prior to the oedipal stage—but even that may not be entirely accurate, or may be in danger of being wrongly applied if our categorization is not differentiated and defined further. In this chapter, I attempt to use the four psychologies as a basis for such differentiation. Here I shall merely sketch out and illustrate the general argument, but I shall continue the discussion in greater detail in chapter 10 with regard to the specific problem of early ego defect.

In the "Three Essays on the Theory of Sexuality," Freud wrote:

> It has justly been said that the oedipus complex is the nuclear complex of the neuroses, and constitutes the essential part of their content. It represents the peak of infantile sexuality, which, through its aftereffects, exercises a decisive influence on the sexuality of adults. Every new arrival on this planet is faced by the task of mastering the oedipus complex; anyone who fails to do so falls a victim to neurosis. With the progress of psychoanalytic studies the importance of the oedipus complex has become more and more clearly evident; its recognition has become the shibboleth that distinguishes the adherents of psychoanalysis from its opponents. (1905, p. 226, fn. added 1920)

In light of such a powerful statement, it is no wonder that the oedipus complex remains central in psychoanalytic theories of pathogenesis. And no wonder that other contributions to pathogenesis are often positioned in relation to the oedipus complex (that is, preoedipal) rather than named in themselves. But Freud's view is limited by, and must reflect in part, the discoveries of his own self-analysis, the culture of his time and, more specifically, the particular patient population seen in (and seen as suitable for) psychoanalysis. Additionally, this view reflects the fact that the relatively late developing triangular oedipus complex, when the child is already verbal, is more available to the light of discovery than are the darkness-shrouded earliest preverbal years that center on one-person (the own body) and two-person (infant and mother) psychologies.

Of course the oedipus complex is of great importance. The biological facts of having been born of two parents and of being born as one sex only (in a two-sex world), coupled with the sociopsychological fact of having (ordinarily) been reared by two parents, lead to immensely significant positionings, desirings, and rivalings vis-à-vis the parents in the life and mind of the growing child. And any earlier developing pathology (or any other developmental feature) will inevitably have the stamp of triangular oedipal relations placed upon it as the child carries such inner phenomena along into the oedipal phase, and they will later (in our patients) be reflected in that particular looking glass. But the very concept of preoedipal pathology grants recognition to the idea that the oedipus complex is but one of the centers of pathogenesis—perhaps it is especially the center in what we call the neuroses—but not necessarily the main center in all persons. By clinical experience and personal history different theorists have become differentially sensitive to varying aspects of the early developmental situation and its role in pathogenesis and have given us the tools for wider formulation.

The most straightforward use of the term *preoedipal pathology* is in relation to phenomena within the domain of the drive psychology—phenomena that we conceptualize as belonging to the libidinal/psychosexual line of development and that culminate in the oedipal constellation—but nonetheless preceding that major flowering of the oedipal phase. These are ordinarily discussed under the paired rubrics fixation and regression. That is, we believe that, sometimes, pleasure and/or distress around phenomena of feeding, bowel function (and the sadomasochistic urges that accompany it), or early fantasies regarding gender identity and sex differences are so great that the stage is set for ready regression from the anxieties of the oedipal period to such domains of earlier fixation.

At times the oedipal triangle seems to take the form of rivalry for feeding and passive care; or for messing, controlling, and sadomasochistic interactions together; or for exhibitionistically showing one's prowess or beauty. That is, presumably earlier psychosexual issues are lived out in the triangular child-mother-father relationships. In other situations we understand that the feared or imagined loss of the penis, or the nonattainment of the oedipal love object, is experienced in terms parallel to earlier loss—say, of breast or feces. And in yet other patients we understand that the identifications that grow out of apparent oedipal-level conflicts are in fact based on those elements of the child-parent interaction that carry along the wishes and failures of earlier psychosexual periods. I think, for example, of a five-year-old boy, never bowel trained, whose intertwined relationships with his parents centered on soiling, but whose parents themselves showed problems in relation to bowel and/or bladder control in their histories *and* in their current functioning. The lines between anal and oedipal interactions, and between object relation and identification, were obscure indeed. Let me give a brief, not atypical, example of preoedipal pathology within the libidinal line of development as it unfolded in the course of an analysis.

ORAL PHASE PATHOLOGY

The patient, Ms. H, sought analysis in her mid-thirties when she moved out of her parents' home for the first time to live with a female friend. This was part of an attempt to begin her life anew; consistent with this wish, she enrolled in classes at a local university to complete her college education at night while she worked during the day. The combined moves forward— moving out and pursuing her education—were followed by intense experiences of anxiety, rage, and depression, the last sufficient to cause her to remain home alone in her apartment, without even getting dressed, on many a weekend. (Her roommate stayed with her own male friend on weekends.) At other times she went out with men—many men—and worried about her promiscuity, but also felt driven by the need for tactile contact. She eventually dropped out of school.

As the analysis proceeded, oedipal issues became paramount in the work. Rivalrous competition with her mother in part underlay her anxiety about success in her education; success would bring her closer to her father, a man with some academic credentials. Sexual relations were seen to have aspects of oedipal victory as well as of fantasied "whorish" power in which she was the active, masculine one, on top, with a penis. The unfolding life history revealed a home with highly seductive (though never explicitly acted upon) relationships with each of her two brothers (one older, one younger)— initiated by the older one toward her, by her toward the younger one—

always characterized by a naivete on her part that allowed her to "inno-cently" go along, to say yes via her naivete without ever consenting to any-thing. This was repeated, later, in relations with other men and in the transference. I do not wish to focus on this material here. Suffice it to say that it was extensively elaborated in fantasy, in action, in the transference, and in the life history and remained a major and productive center of the analytic work from start to finish.

But it was never the full story. Content suggestive of early oral issues was al-ways there alongside the oedipal material—sometimes in alternation, some-times with a sense of simultaneity. I recall, in many a session, wondering toward which of the two simultaneously unfolding levels an interpretation might best be addressed in order to reach the patient in her most central im-mediate experience. Thus, fellatio as an important form of sexual pleasure was often connected with fantasies of incorporation of the penis and wishes to make up for imagined castration, but at other times to "fill me up" via men (father) as "my mother never did." Bouts of nausea in sexual contacts that, for her, had an aura of connectedness to her brothers or father eventually disap-peared with interpretation of the incestuous fantasies, but nausea associated with fellatio as a means of "filling [her] up" remained for a time after that, and eventually was understood to connect to the sense of the "bad" things that she had taken in from mother. Separations came to be understood both as losses of father to mother (for example, when I went away the patient was particularly distraught over her idea that it was with my wife), but also, and eventually far more powerfully, as losses of mother herself. This latter mirrored actual sepa-rations of her very early years, and emotional unavailability of mother as a chronic state, and produced intense longings.

Other material, too, pointed in both directions—at times to oedipal phase issues and at times to early oral issues. To have a boyfriend shielded her, she felt, from seduction by and of me; but being with him (like the tactile com-fort she sought in her first year living away from her parental home) was like "being covered by a warm blanket"—an experience she came to feel in rela-tion to my voice as the analysis progressed. Also, wishes to have a baby emerged with great force. In fantasy, it would be her baby with her father, the proof of her oedipal victory. But it, too, like the incorporated penis, would make her feel "filled"; with the baby inside she would be feeding her-self by feeding it; and she would be a better mother to the baby and to herself than her mother had been. And one last illustration of the two-sidedness of the material: the patient had been hypnotized in a classroom demonstration while in high school. A powerful and exciting fantasy developed after that of being enslaved (hypnotized) by one of her brothers, drawn to him by his seductiveness, controlled by him. But much later, her fear of being "enslaved" by her own longings for maternal care (felt largely in the transference) emerged with great force and clarity.

During the course of the work, the sense of a sickly, weepy early childhood emerged with, as noted, separations from mother in the earliest years. The patient was a thumbsucker. She recalled loving the touch of her mother's silky nightgown, and then tactile contact altogether. She recalled singing herself to sleep, self-soothing, to fill the experienced void left by her emotionally absent mother. She recalled a sense of the mother's (oral) neediness, a sense that she would be "sucked into" her mother to meet the mother's need for her. Faulty early object relationships can leave one or another of an endless array of marks on the personality. In this instance, and the part that I am particularly choosing to emphasize here, there was a lasting sense of a deep oral hunger, a need for contact, soothing, and "filling."

At times in the analysis, the oral-phase issues served as a regressive defense against oedipal issues. At times, however, the reverse seemed to be the case, oedipal desires used to defend against oral longings. Progressively, as the analysis went on, the oral phase issues were seen as a center of pathological organization in their own right—with longings, fantasies, avoidances, and self-perpetuating conflict centered on them. These conflicts and wishes in fact gave shape to much of the oedipal material—the preference for fellatio and the fantasies of oedipal victory through incorporation, now of the penis, now of a baby.

Ms. H gives us one kind of example of "preoedipal" pathology— primary oral phase disturbance followed by, combined with, shaping, and also regressively defending against oedipal phase pathology. This is preoedipal within the conceptual framework of the psychosexual/drive/ oedipal line of development. But it is not my sense that this is the most usual situation in which the concept preoedipal pathology is invoked. More often the term *preoedipal pathology* is used to refer to disturbances that are connected, in my terms, to the psychologies of ego, object relations, and self. In this usage, the term *preoedipal* is used out of conceptual habit in a way. It actually refers to *earlier*-than-oedipal pathology, but in *different regions* of the personality. Its relation to oedipal pathology is less clear than that of pathology of earlier psychosexual phases. Referring to this pathology merely as preoedipal fails to give it the degree of conceptual differentiation which our theories are now capable of providing. I want to turn to some instances of such pathology now.

In describing instances of pathology related to separation-individuation, internalized object relations, self experience, and aspects of faulty ego development (the last in chapter 10), I do not mean to imply that these are separate from one another or from drive experiences. But I have tried to se- lect instances where the balance is more one way than another, where the disturbance is probably early in origin but where a significant aspect of its or- ganization is productively seen in terms of self (boundaries or esteem), in- ternalized object relations, or ego defect.

SEPARATION-INDIVIDUATION

A patient, Ms. I, came to treatment reporting that "I disappear," that she has had this experience for years, and that she wanted help with it because she had a vague fear that it would get worse after her child was born (she was several months pregnant with her first child). Her description of "disappear- ing" was obscure and fragmentary and her general state panic-ridden, but she was articulate, intelligent, and highly motivated. I began to work with some hesitation, on a trial basis, but it rapidly became clear that she could work reliably and well, and we began a three times weekly intensive psycho- therapy that continued for several years. Gradually, it became clear that states of "disappearing" involved severe anxiety attacks associated with vary- ing mental contents, any of which could loosely fit under the concept of dis- appearing. Thus, she would feel "lost in a forest, wandering, totally alone," or she would feel "pulled as though by a magnet, unable to wrench free." These were vague contents; my putting them into (even the patient's) words makes them sound more precise than they ever were. At times these states sounded like depersonalization or derealization experiences, in varying pro- portions between the two. The patient never did recall when and why she started referring to these states as disappearing.

One of a pair of twins, she remembers being the one who insisted on same- ness, loyalty, being together with her twin sister. Other memories existed side by side, however; she was ornery, willful, stubborn, would not ever stand corrected, held on to individualized fantasies of a great future for herself, herself alone. But even more striking than the sibling twinship in her revelation of her history was the "twinship" she had with her mother—and there are external factors corroborating this as (at least in part, probably large part) a reality. The two of them were extraordinarily close, and the patient recalled "wooing" her mother into a special relationship that excluded her twin sister. Additionally, the generational distinction was unstable. That is, at times the mother was a super-available mother, meeting every need, catering to every whim of the patient (as a young girl); at other times she was like another sister, apparently identified with this child. Ms. I, in her twenties, married, and living far from her mother and sister when I began to work with her, carried the sense of the dual twinships within her. She let me know in no uncertain terms that nothing would break up her relationship to her mother, indeed that I could not even expect that she would speak to me as openly as she did to her. (She did seem to speak with astonishing openness to her, and the mother's responses seemed to be totally nonjudgmental, accepting.)

This all changed to a very considerable degree over a treatment of several years' duration. I wish to focus on just four features of the patient that became clear as the work went on.

The first two are reciprocals in a sense, two contrasting yet linked sides of the symptom "disappearing." It became clear that the experience of disappearing would come when she started feeling too close to her family-of-childhood, either in thought or in actuality. The way I saw it, and the interpretation that I offered, which seemed to match her history, her description of her symptom, and the precipitating event, was that the closeness made her fear a loss of her very selfness, the self that she had won only with great difficulty. That is, she feared disappearing into her sibling/self and mother/self unities. But the other, reciprocal, precipitant (each occurring many times before we were able to grasp it in some way), was when she felt a powerful sense of individuality and success in her career. (She was a business executive of considerable influence.) Here the interpretation offered focused on the defensive aspects of disappearing—that is, *giving up* the achieved individuality and success in order to hold on to the sense of connectedness with her sister and her mother. That is, she made her strong and independent self "disappear" to fulfill the wish not to feel too separated from one or the other of the unities. From both sides, she seemed to be dealing with *boundary* issues—too close or too distant each precipitating a sense of loss of herself. The two primary initial descriptions of her states of disappearing—being drawn as though to a magnet (on the one hand) or lost in a forest alone (on the other)—seem to reflect the two opposite poles of absorption and of too much independence, each of which precipitated disappearances.

It seemed consistent during the treatment that a third aspect of this patient's functioning was her adamant refusal (in general) to receive transference interpretations. Though these were offered, the patient was intolerant of them. She would, not completely figuratively, rear up like a cornered cat and claw her way free if the therapist put himself into her thoughts. It was clear that this, too, was a boundary issue. The therapist was "the doctor." He should stay in his place, not in her head. We learned to get around this in ways, when more trust developed, but even then it was mainly the stubborn, willful, individualistic side of her that, transferentially, formed the relationship to the therapist. And this was an aspect of her early (and current) struggle against loss of individuality. But the alliance with the therapist was very strong and reliable; there, the therapist was another person, in his place, and that, in itself, was experienced as therapeutic by her.

The fourth feature I wish to mention dates from something we learned about her adolescence. Just at the time when her panic states began, this budding adolescent, alive with her own sexuality, chanced to discover her father in an extramarital affair. Suddenly this sexually admired man was *too* sexual for the young adolescent girl. She turned from him, and back to her sister/mother twinship, and her symptom began. Just as Greenson (1967) and Stoller (1968) have written of the boy's relation to the early father that helps promote a "disidentification" from mother, so too can the male play this role for the early adolescent girl—helping her out of the reactivated intense relation to the mother-of-infancy. But this went awry here—perhaps too easily, given the patient's leaning in the direction of the regressive move to mother in any event. Eventually I came to understand this aspect of the patient's conflict as the plight of being caught "between the devil and the deep blue sea." That phrase came to have great meaning. Having seen the same constellation in a second patient, of course with individual life-historical differences in the details, I now see that phrase as capturing something that is a significant developmental plight for some individuals. The father was the devil of sexuality. The mother was the deep blue sea—linked to Freud's (1930) "oceanic" feeling—the mother of union, loss of self, disappearance. For Ms. I, her fantasies regarding her father, the (sexual) devil, were too much for her to cope with, and she drifted back to the deep blue sea—her ever available mother, absorption, and disappearance. Thus began a lifelong struggle over the wish for and fear of merger. (Another of my patients, in a similar plight, "chose" the devil—the father not only rescuing her from her own and mother's pull toward merger but also providing the warmth that the sought after union with the cold mother could not provide.)

Late in the treatment, when associations to a dream led to a reconstruction of much of this material for the patient, she recalled efforts to get close to her father as a child, but also of certain actions by her mother in response which "pulled me back, as though to a magnet."

I came to understand the material with Ms. I as showing pathological resolution of issues of separation-individuation and attendant problems of self and object formation. In the terms that I am using in this book, I see her pathology as involving both failures in the formation of the boundaries of the self and distortions of internalized object relations, wherein her mother/sister/self equivalences in her mind remained a prominent, though pathological, form of her self experience. But note that issues of drive—that is, of intense and ongoing sexual fantasy in relation to her father—are not absent from the particular constellation of separation-individuation issues seen here. I am not arguing for exclusivity; drive, ego, object relations, and self formations are in all of us, however we are organized inside; but separation-individuation issues were at the center of her personal hierarchy. This patient reveals preoedipal pathology only in the sense of earlier than oedipal (or, at least, I believe the problems had their start in the first two years of life). It is of equal importance to recognize that it is in another sense *non*oedipal—that is, in a different developmental region. Though a successful oedipal tie to her father might have pulled her out of her pathological twinship relationships and fantasies, I do not believe the pathology is best viewed as the result of regression from oedipal conflict. Instead, I see it as primary.

INTERNALIZED OBJECT RELATIONS

Dr. J, a forty-seven-year-old physician, entered analysis because of problems in his relationships with women. He regularly met new women whom he admired greatly, but soon found himself in relations with them of a profoundly attacking quality—nasty, degrading, and with fantasies (never acted upon) of physical abuse as well. His relations with colleagues were characterized by hate-filled envy, distrust, and fear of being "attacked" in the arena of his professional functioning (where he actually did rather well). He was an only child, and I later learned that hate-filled, abusive relationships were also present among his mother, his father, and himself.

The transference that was rapidly established seemed to be oedipal in quality—with both positive and negative oedipal elements. The patient experienced himself as winning out over other (especially male) patients in pleasing and fascinating the analyst-as-mother. And in counterpoint, the patient had homosexual fantasies of analyst-like figures with whom he could leave behind all women. A central aspect of the remembered content of his life had similarities to this. He had vivid recall of being on a summer camping trip with an uncle and aunt and regularly overhearing sexual relations between them; he noticed that his aunt always seemed glowing and tender on the morning after. Soon thereafter he transposed this event onto his parents and became preoccupied with the idea that in their sexual relationship his father really made his mother happy, "glowing." He then developed two fantasies: of being with his mother sexually and making her as happy as his father made her (in his imagination), and of being with his father sexually and being made that happy by him. These were the two fantasies that colored the transference.

That much was clear, but nothing else seemed to fit: the cruel hatefulness that characterized his relations with women and colleagues (and that regularly spilled over into the relation to the analyst), his tendency to fall asleep instantly in the sessions when his obvious anger at the analyst was noted, and a history of violent physical and verbal abuse among the members of his family were all at odds with the beatific images of glowing sexuality. His earliest "memory" was of his father "trying to kill me" out of envious rage for the attention he as a child received from his mother, and of his mother cursing and throwing things at his father in retaliation. The sorting out of the realities, projections, and identifications in this "memory" was an endless process. But all of the evidence seemed to be that destructive and hate-filled physical violence characterized the family relationships from the patient's earliest months. Given this history, his fantasy of his mother's postsexual bliss was understood to be necessary to him; it came to exist side by side with fantasies of sex as violence, and (dynamically) came to be used as an idealizing reversal of the remembered hate-filled relations within the family.

The understanding that was eventually arrived at was that early, physically abusive, hate-filled internalized object relations persisted and dominated the psychopathology. These were partially split off (hence his falling asleep at their mention) and partially enacted (with women and colleagues). The idealization that was experienced in meeting new women, in a central aspect of the relation to the analyst, and in the fantasies regarding his parents' blissful sexual relations, were the other side of the coin. But these served primarily in denial and splitting off, helping him preserve a feeling of worth.

In the terms I am using in this book, pathological early internalized object relations were at the core of the disturbance, making it such that the "oedipal" resolution (fantasies of parental bliss, and of his bliss with one or the other of them) was thoroughly unstable, even unreal—contradicted by the ongoing familial realities and serving mostly as a fragile, denying, idealization, buttressing him against the inner flooding of hate. Here, though, in contrast to the previous patient (Ms. I) who was almost totally unable to use her relation to her father to pull herself out of excessive merger with her mother and sister, this man did use images of blissful sexuality to cover over hate-filled preoccupations and memories. But, although they involve mother, father, and self and are thus triangular, and although they involve overheard sexual activity, the primary quality he extracted from these memories was their beatific nature—because that is what he needed in his effort to remedy the primary area of pathology: destructive, hate- and envy-filled internalized images of human connectedness. Such pathology, too, is preoedipal (that is, early), but it is better described in terms of an other-than-oedipal developmental line; here the pathology is laid down in terms of destructive internalized object relations.

SELF EXPERIENCE

The last patient whose analysis I wish to discuss here is one already described in the previous chapter: Mr. E. But I wish to use the material this time to make an additional point. In the preceding three examples, my point was that preoedipal pathology can take quite different forms and is better described in more differentiated ways—as pathology of early psychosexual phases or as pathology of self and object (illustrated by one patient with separation-individuation disturbances and another with pathological internalized object representations and relations). With Mr. E, I wish to consider that not all pathology in the other-than-oedipal area—that is, not all self or object pathology—need be primarily *preoedipal* (and see my discussion of Joan Fleming's [1975] case in chapter 10).

I have already discussed Mitchell's (1984) concept of the "developmental tilt"—that is, the idea that other-than-oedipal sources of pathology are generally seen as earlier than oedipal and as having no real contributory significance in the oedipal and postoedipal period. His point was that by contrast to this view, object relational issues are significant throughout the life cycle. My own attempt in chapter 4 was to expand his point and argue that phenomena in each of the regions of drive, ego, object relations, and self contain very early (preoedipal) core developments which can go wrong (creating a center of pathology) and which in the normal case must undergo various developments if optimal growth and function are to be achieved. On the other hand, I also suggested that phenomena in the domains of drive, ego, object relations, and self have significant aspects that continue to develop postoedipally.

To my surprise at times, as Mr. E's analysis proceeded, I regularly found that a particular experience of self, his "needy/awful" feeling, continued to command center stage. Though sometimes we saw its position in the oedipal constellation and at other times we saw its defensive function in relation to sexuality and anger, as these issues became clear they did not replace that central self experience in importance. Much of significance was learned about those other areas, and yet, each time, those problems would fade into the background—as though less urgent—and the self experience again would assume centrality, leading us into yet another area of productive work. But, and here is my point, through it all, and in spite of pathology centered around a particular experience of self, it never seemed to me that what we were working with had very early, primarily preoedipal, origins. Mr. E, indeed, seemed to me quite an intact individual—basically sound in those core domains that we look to in assessment of psychological stability; he had stable and emotionally meaningful object relations, access to at least a fair array of his emotions, a reliable set of, for him, characteristic modes of defense, the capacity for modulated impulse expression, and tools of affect modulation, thought, speech, judgment, and insight ready to be used. He was, incidentally, quite capable of love, work, and play—even at the start of his analysis. And yet he suffered significantly. He carried with him a painful inner experience that was a spoiler of innumerable facets of, and moments in, his life.

My impression is that the relationship to his father (and in secondary ways to his mother as well), a relationship of "nonrecognition" and of treating him like an object to be ignored or used, a relationship continuing in the form of "strain trauma" (Kris, 1956a) all through his childhood and early adolescence, was destructive of his inner experience of self—and had its main destructive force in a cumulative way precisely because of its continuance in the long period of childhood and adolescence. Far be it for me to say, and nor is it necessary for me to argue, that there were no seeds of this early on. But my best understanding of the patient was that it was the *continued* (postoedipal) destructive impact of the father's ignoring and using him that had the primary and cumulative pathogenic effect.

I am not here saying that what is pathogenic postoedipally need come only from the outside. The basic stance of the analytic work with Mr. E was an intrapsychic one, and our focus was on the overdetermination and multiple functions of this inner self experience. This stance eventuated in our understanding of his fantasies about, his characterological adaptations to, and his defensive, expressive, and repetitious uses of an experience *begun* in the actual father-son relationship but then elaborated intrapsychically. But the central pathogenic role of events in the mid-childhood through early adolescent years remained in the forefront.

I certainly do not feel that the evidence for such later developing pathology is clearly in, and in fact I myself would have strong doubts about that view in general, if not linked to early seeds. Nonetheless, I think it is worth considering that the concept of preoedipal pathology errs not only in failing to distinguish among clinically differentiable phenomena in the domains of ego, self, and object relations early on, but also in the often implicit assumption that phenomena partially or more fully outside of the libidinal drive/ defense/superego line of development necessarily have their impact earlier than the oedipal phase. As I suggested in chapter 4, I believe that much of what we later see as pathological repetition of old object relationships reflects chronic experiences of the elementary-school age—the mid-childhood—years. This so-called latency period is (relatively) latent only with respect to drive phenomena, but hardly at all with respect to the internalization of the experienced field of object relations, and with that, of characteristic defenses.

In overview, then, I suggest that the term *preoedipal pathology* is often used loosely in the literature as though it refers to one large undifferentiated array. This is so, I believe, because of the historical development of psychoanalytic theory (wherein the oedipus complex was at the center) and continuing debates about the relative centrality of that set of issues. But I believe that we can make significant conceptual differentiations within the domain of preoedipal pathology which can help us in our clinical work. I have tried to do that in this chapter: to clarify the concept of preoedipal pathology and to show that, in doing so, it is useful to keep in mind the several psychologies (drive, ego, object relations, self) that psychoanalysis has produced. Early pathology can form in any of those domains, and so our view of what is preoedipal has to be broad enough to encompass all of them. We are actually talking, of course, simply about *early* pathological development, and it is merely an anachronism—growing out of the historical development of psychoanalysis and the historical precedence of our understanding of oedipal pathology—that we use *preoedipal* (rather than simply *early*) to position ourselves in this domain.

I have not yet discussed early pathology in the domain of the psychology of the ego, and I shall turn to that topic in the next chapter.

CHAPTER 10

The Concept of Ego Defect

IN PART I, I introduced a perhaps deceptively simple set of propositions. I suggested that the adult (and even the child) has tools for adaptation, reality testing, and defense that the infant does not yet have in full measure and that, therefore, these must have developed in the time between infancy and childhood or adulthood. I added that anything that thus develops can develop poorly or well; and I proposed thinking of those poor (failed or aberrant) developments in the spheres of adaptation, reality testing, and defense as ego defects. In the present chapter, I would like to expand these propositions in a number of directions.

I am not here discussing, say, *experiences* of "emptiness" (Singer, 1988) or a *sense* of defect (Coen, 1986); of course those subjective states have to be analyzed before one can say anything intelligent about them in any individual instance. But this differs from a judgment that often it is the analyst who makes regarding some inadequately developed tool of psychic functioning—a judgment that equally often the patient shares, or has been telling the analyst about in one way or another all along.

I shall begin with an introductory discussion of the range of the problem under consideration and then turn to a clinical presentation of four cases— two that I am personally familiar with and two from the published literature.

INTRODUCTORY CONSIDERATIONS

Concern with the question of ego defect is certainly not new. Freud (1937) explored the question as part of his paper on the interminability of psychoanalysis. It is certainly also a part of what Balint (1968) was pursuing in his writings on the basic fault. And child analysts, perhaps closer in time to the site of those developmental failures, have not failed to give recognition to them (Alpert, 1959; Redl, 1951; Weil, 1953, 1956). Anna Freud (1974) discusses it most extensively:

> What we have been most familiar with in the analytic literature so far are the abnormalities caused by the incidence of trauma, and of conflict between the internal agencies followed by anxiety, defense, and compromise formation. What have received much less attention and are added here are the defects in the personality structure itself which are caused by the aforementioned developmental irregularities and failures. We can thus differentiate between two types of infantile psychopathology. The one based on conflict is responsible for the anxiety states, and the phobic, hysterical, and obsessional manifestations, i.e., the infantile neuroses; the one based on developmental defects, for the psychosomatic symptomatology, the backwardness, the atypical and borderline states.
>
> It would be convenient to take the point of view that success or failure on the developmental lines primarily shapes the personalities which secondarily become involved in internal conflict. But any statement of this kind would be a gross falsification once the infant ceases to be an undifferentiated, unstructured being. It would ignore the temporal relations between the two processes which occur simultaneously, not subsequent to each other. Progress on the [developmental] lines is interfered with constantly by conflict, repression, and consequent regression, while the conflicts themselves and quite especially the meth-

ods available for their solution are wholly dependent on the shape and
level of personal development which has been reached.

However different in origins the two types of psychopathology are,
in the clinical picture they are totally intertwined, a fact which ac-
counts for their usually being treated as one. (pp. 70–71)

But the recent stir in the psychoanalytic literature in relation to the concept of *defect* really spills over from arguments regarding Kohut's (1971,
1977) work on the different—but easily confused—concept of *deficit*. I
propose distinguishing the two as follows. A deficit (in parallel to not having enough money in the bank) involves an *insufficiency of input* from the
surround—ordinarily from the primary caretakers. A defect, by contrast,
refers to something that is not working well (in parallel to something being
broken); it is within the person (not the surround), *by whatever means it
got there*.

In his discussions, Kohut emphasized deficiencies in two areas in particular: insufficient "mirroring" of the child (with its consequences for primary
self feeling, self worth, and the experience of oneself as a center of initiative,
an active agent) and the provision of insufficient opportunity for the child to
idealize the parent(s) (with its consequences for both the formation and the
taming of goals, values, and ideals). But surely these are not the only significant and potential deficiencies in parental input. All of the basic achievements going into what (in chapter 4) I described as the construction of an
intrapsychic life require some optimal participation from the primary
caretaker—whether merely the general assistance provided by their facilitating environment (Winnicott, 1965) or more specific acts and inputs that
provide the basis for identification and other forms of learning. Perhaps we
can understand Kohut's contribution to be a clarification of the necessary
inputs (and the related deficiencies or deficits) for the optimal development
of the narcissistic sector of the personality. But other inputs (and their related deficiencies) are critical to the formation of impulse control, affect tolerance, the expansion of the affect array, development of a stable array of
defenses, and the moves toward trust, toward signal anxiety, and toward
object constancy—to name just a few.

Kohut's writings created the stir they did in part because they shook up
comfortable beliefs regarding some areas of pathology and technique, but
also because they seemed to go so far in locating the source of pathology in

the failed parental inputs—something that seemed regressive in terms of the whole conceptual achievement of psychoanalysis over the years. So narcissistic pathology (or was it *all* pathology in the "superordinate" conception of the Self? [Kohut, 1977]) looked too much like a deficiency disease, without sufficient recognition of (a) internal elaboration and (b) primary sources (for example, the drives and the consequences of coping with them) within the developing person. A closely related argument is over the techniques advanced by Kohut, which include a heavy dose of developmental facilitation through the provision of an empathic surround and an understanding acceptance—albeit in the context of our usual quiet listening and interpretive work.

Defect is a very different concept. I do not doubt for a moment that deficits, as I have just defined them, exist and have an impact. Quite the reverse; I believe they are significant far beyond the sphere (the narcissistic sector) that Kohut addresses. But *defect* says that something has not developed well. Nothing is said about the source of the failure or aberration of development. It could stem from a deficit—that is, a deficient input in some area. For example, reliable parental care ordinarily produces the capacity for trust and hence delay (as will be discussed); a *deficit* in such reliable care might therefore produce a *defect* in the capacity for delay. Or a defect could stem from some inborn biological condition, or trauma, or early pain and illness (see Chethik, 1984; Pine, 1986a) that makes an ordinary parental provision insufficient in this particular instance. Or it could stem from early conflict resolutions that have the effect of stunting ego development (producing "defects") in one or another area (see my [Pine, 1974] description of the developmental consequences of an early solution through pseudoimbecility, and Joseph Youngerman's [1979] description of a parallel effect of an early solution through mutism). But in each of these instances—whatever the source—the residue is some significant failure in the development of an aspect of ego function: of adaptation, reality testing, and/or defense.

Such defects are certainly not independent of conflict. Not only may they have resulted from the workings of conflict but—whatever their source—they will become caught up in intrapsychic experience, in the responses of others, in self perceptions and, through these, work their way into fantasy and get conflictual wishes attached to them. They will achieve psychic representation and be treated like any mental content—that is, subject to conflictual elaborations. To take a gross example, blindness—a biological

defect—will not fail to take on psychic meaning and be conflictually elaborated. But the very fact that defects are thus tied up with conflict may, I believe, at times blind us to the defect aspect—because one more, and then
again still one more, interpretation of a conflictual derivative or source will
forever be possible, and may result in a failure to give recognition to the fact
of a defect with whatever implications for technique (if any) that fact may
have. (The reverse problem may also come up; that is, the fact of a defect
can blind one to its conflictual elaborations that require interpretation.)

Let me try to give a sense of the array of defects that may occur in the
course of development and in the context of failures of adequate care from
the surround. I emphasize *adequate* care; early illness, or low thresholds and
hyperreactivity in the child, for example, may render otherwise adequate
care less than adequate—making it such that it fails to comfort, or inducing
stress in the caretaker that undercuts and distorts the caretaking acts. But, in
any event, many developments can go wrong.

What are some of those features of ego function that must develop and
that therefore can develop poorly? Anna Freud (1965), in attempting to arrive at modes of assessing normality and pathology in children, and noting
that development continually leads to shifts in the specifics of what we actually see, proposed assessing four general characteristics of the child. These
characteristics, she felt, had some predictive power regarding how well the
child was likely to develop henceforth. Three of those that she described,
sublimation potential, frustration tolerance, and the *attitude to anxiety*, are
the kinds of developmental features that I have in mind. If they develop well,
they serve as positive resources for subsequent development. If they develop
poorly, however, they can lead to mushrooming difficulties—to problems in
coping with the ongoing and inevitable stresses in relation to urges, object
relations, and self experiences.

Let me develop a considerably larger list. The developmental pie can be
sliced in many ways, and there is nothing sacred about the particular order
or groupings that I shall now give. Additionally, all of what follows is
necessarily conjectural, because the construction of modes of functioning is
not something that we hear in the content of fantasies or can directly observe. But the outcomes of such faulty ego construction are endemic in our
patients.

To begin with, *trust* is crucial. It is generally assumed to develop when
early needs (hunger especially, but also warmth, rocking, relief from excess

stimulation) are reliably met by the significant caretaker, such that the infant can come to expect the cycle: need → satisfaction (or relief). That expectation of relief or satisfaction *is* what we refer to as trust. Such experiences also provide the first experiential glue of connection to the object. Additionally, such trust allows *delay* in the face of need (because satisfaction comes to be expected); and in these moments of delay—as in contented and quiescent, but wakeful, periods altogether—much of learning takes place. Here, then, are some of the beginnings of early learning and inner modulation—that is, of aspects of ego functioning. The reverse, constant nonsatisfaction in the face of need, also leads to learning, but in this case learning that nonsatisfaction and the escalation of distress is what is to be expected. But that is precisely the sort of malformation—affecting the earliest qualities of self experience, of object relation, and of the predictable and quiescent versus stressed and chaotic organization of experience—that I mean to highlight. It can be seen as preoedipal pathology in the ego domain or, as I prefer, as a defect in ego development.

This leads naturally into discussion of the conditions for the development of *signal* versus *panic anxiety*, or gradations in between. When need (whether for nursing, or for other object contact, or a responsive confirming look or smile, or for stimulation) is regularly followed by nonsatisfaction, then all that the need comes to signal, so to speak, is the continuance or exacerbation of distress. In such a case, distress escalates to panic rapidly, without the intervention of reliable defenses. The move to true signal anxiety takes place when, in the face of need and in the reliable expectation of relief, there can be delay of the escalation of distress and anxiety and the gradual emergence of higher-order modes of coping. Subsequently, the first distress can signal the potential of greater distress and set now available defenses in operation.

Another way to describe these early events is in terms of the beginnings of *internal self-regulation*. For the infant who comes to expect satisfaction and/or relief, that very expectation is already a regulator of inner state. The infant who wakes and looks around, or later babbles and coos, or finds a thumb and sucks, or rocks and calls out (trustingly) is, in each case, exercising a form of control, of regulation, in relation to inner experience and can do this because prior experiences have already built in an assurance of satisfaction or relief. By contrast, intense distress or panic can be seen as a failure of internal self-regulation in itself, and also as a state too powerful to be regulated internally once under way, or finally as a state of cognitive confusion (because of affect flooding) in which learnings and actions relevant to self-regulation are unlikely to occur. We know that individuals differ, later on, in terms of their tendency to achieve self-regulation via alcohol or other drugs or via addictive relationships or magical expectations of others, or in the degree to which they give up in despair in the face of distress, or spill it out into action or diffuse affective outbursts. While surely not hardened in concrete in the earliest months, it seems not unlikely that the beginnings of these failures of self-regulation occur in the infant in some such ways as I have attempted to describe. But if this is the case, then the child meets susbsequent experience already handicapped, and the failures mount.

Such early phenomena may also have a role in the formation of another core difference that we see later on—in the basic *attitude toward one's impulses* as ego alien and threatening or as acceptable and susceptible to modification. There is no question that this is a striking difference in people who come for analysis later on, with variation across the full range. Urges that can be tolerated to robust degrees and described reasonably comfortably by some are fearfully evaded and denied by others. This is not to say that an apparent tolerance of urges may not itself at times cover unconscious guilt, or be a form of narcissistic exhibitionism—that is, be itself an aspect of the particular pathology—but nonetheless I believe profound variation along this dimension to be fairly obvious in the array of patients seen by any one of us, and we generally view tolerance of impulse life (in the context of a reasonably well organized personality) as a positive resource. I would conjecture that early experiences of reliable relief, coupled with reassuring or playful parental attitudes toward the urge experience and its bodily expressions (such as hunger, defecation), as well as the fact that moments of such urge and bodily need can be (for some) nodal points for satisfying infant-caretaker interactions altogether—that all of these set the groundwork for a more comfortable attitude toward one's bodily functions and sensations, and the wishful urges derived from them. Conversely, nonsatisfaction and mounting distress, parental discomfort and anxiety in the face of such experiences, and the consequent negative infant-caretaker moments in relation to them can begin the formation of attitudes in which urges are, by experience and by identification, seen in negative terms by the infant—and later on as ego alien and threatening. Of course, even in the positive experiences, guilt and anxiety may change the attitude toward impulses as conflictual fantasies develop around them; on the other hand, such good early experiences of urge and response to them may be among the forerunners of lesser severity of superego function.

Another feature of early development that can proceed for good or for ill is what I shall refer to as the *patterning of libidinal need*. When urges are routinely unsatisfied, or inconsistently or conflictually satisfied, they cannot fall into place, in reliable and patterned ways and in object-related terms—which patterning would itself serve as a building block for later adaptation and higher-order functioning. In the optimally developing child, step-by-step, phase-by-phase, higher-level need states are encountered and patterns of defense (in relation to the urge) and gratification (in relation to the object) are developed. Sandler and Sandler (1978) have convincingly argued that anticipated role relationships come to be part of wishes (wished-for patterns of interaction). This contributes to the binding together of self and object in patterns of reliable satisfaction. Such reliable satisfactions are core phenomena binding together (giving continuity and cohesion to) the self experience as well, and additionally enhancing self-esteem. At the opposite extreme, urges become intrusive stimuli from within—or actually, remain such. Winnicott (1960a) describes how, early on, urges are experienced as external—"like a clap of thunder or a hit" (p. 141)—a quality that alters (and leads to "ownership" of urges) when satisfaction comes. The absence of such achievements deprives the person of a solid base for subsequent adaptation, instead leaving a further adaptational demand—that of coping with intrusive inner (drive) stimuli. Libidinal urges can then be problematic in two central ways: their failed role as the glue of object relations and self experience because of developmental failures, and their presence as tormenting and intrusive inner stimuli adding to the stimulus barrage. Naturally, this is not either-or, but I am trying to highlight significant early variations among individuals that affect their capacity to master later demands.

Variations in *frustration tolerance* result from and subsequently affect all of these early developments as well. This is a critical aspect of what I described earlier in terms of the development of delay, when satisfaction or relief can be reliably expected. Naturally the development of frustration tolerance is overdetermined—with contributions as least from the side of constitutional threshold factors, early familial identifications, and early experiences with satisfaction or its absence—but in any case, frustration tolerance/intolerance becomes a critical variable affecting later adaptive capacity.

In many ways, all of the features of early development that I have described thus far (that is, the development of trust, signal anxiety, internal self-regulation, impulse and frustration tolerance, and the patterning of libidinal need) overlap with one another and are discriminable conceptually only to a degree. But another feature of early development which affects later adaptation to the inner and the outer world is relatively more differentiated from those already discussed. I refer to the *activity-passivity balance*. In later life, individuals vary in the degree to which they are psychological "doers." (I do not mean doers in the world outside—"captains of industry" and the like; but rather, initiators rather than reactors, copers rather than absorbers, in the personal inner world.) Many possible early sources of this can be teased out: unknown constitutional factors; early experiences with the summoning of caretakers (the still vague cry for relief) that lead to success and thus continuance of activity (as opposed to nonsuccess leading to despair); early quiescent moments when visual-motor play can take place and the infant can experience himself or herself as a force that can make interesting things happen (in contrast to the absence of these moments when distress-need-anxiety pervades early experience); and early identifications with parental style. But whatever the source, the activity-passivity balance affects subsequent function—probably with excesses in either direction making for difficulty.

Let me mention a few more areas of potential early failure in what we can group as ego functions, each very briefly. The achievement of, or failure to achieve, early *self-other differentiation* is not only (in the instance of failure) a form of ego defect in itself but has consequences for the development of reality testing that are pervasive in their effects. Certainly one of the earliest reality discriminations that must be made is in terms of this distinction between self and other. While it now seems clear that such early discrimination capacities are neurologically built in, affectively significant moments in which there is a "merger" experience contradict the straightforward experience of perceptual discrimination (see chapter 11). The achievement of self-other differentiation that I write of here is the one that takes place against the tide of wished-for-merger in the setting of moments of intensely gratifying "oneness" experience. And the achievement of such a reliable anchoring in reality, against the press of wish, provides a start for all subsequent conquests of the reality principle over the pleasure principle.

The achievement of a *tie between need satisfaction and specific, longed for, others*—and additionally to concern for the object—must be built upon developments already described. In the absence of reliable satisfaction, need becomes or remains desperate, imperious—more important than the specific object; what matters is only the negative need state within and ridding oneself of it. Experiences of reliable gratification plus firm discrimination of self-other boundaries, on the other hand, must contribute to specificity of object ties and concern for the other.

Differentiation of the affect array (Pine, 1979a) is yet another feature of early development with significant consequences for later coping with the inner and outer worlds. Anny Katan (1961) stressed the control possibilities inherent in the naming, hence differentiating, of affects for the child. And more recently Theodore Gaensbauer (1982) has shown the probable precocious differentiation of affect in response to trauma. While it is certainly too early to say how affect differentiation achieved in such contrary ways may affect later functioning, the general fact that such differentiation can play a significant role in optimal functioning seems clear from clinical work.

Self-esteem, having origins in early experiences of self-as-doer (White, 1963; Broucek, 1979; Pine, 1985), in experiences of good internal states, as well as in the reflected glow of parental pleasure in the infant, is yet another early developing feature of intrapsychic experience. In its negative form, it is potentially a center of disturbance in itself as well as an encumbrance to the development of frustration tolerance, of positive relatedness from which subsequent good experiences can be drawn, and of a secure base for the ownership of experience.

The *taming of aggression*, ordinarily occurring in large part through the integration of loving and rageful images of self and other, may be impaired. This happens in part because the degree of reactive rage in the overwhelmed and unsatisfied child is more than can be mastered and in part because the defensive splitting, with object-preservative intent, adds to the problem by preventing the loving images from modifying the hate-filled images as they do in normal development. The resultant love/hate split, or, more typically, idealization/hate split, can be viewed as one more kind of ego defect.

The *maturation of defenses* toward greater flexibility and higher-order forms can be impaired when, in the face of chronic distress and nonsatisfaction, early forming defenses are clung to desperately, even though often unsuccessfully (Pine, 1986a). The periods of ease, of psychic flexibility and play, of relative trust which would allow for a relaxation of guardedness and the taking in or creation of new modes of behaving, intrapsychically and externally, are all too rare and thus is produced the rigid repetition of whatever defensive style has once been lighted upon.

And finally, *sublimation potential* (A. Freud, 1965), derived from whatever early sources, is a profoundly valuable tool for the encounter with later psychological demands—opening up a whole new mode of potential resolution.

This is a fairly extensive list of potential early developments, developments that can go wrong and, in doing so, impair the individual's adaptive, reality testing, or defense capacities—thus creating (in my terms) ego defects. I have been attempting to show possible routes to the development of such developmental defects. Once again, there is no irreconcilability between defects and conflicts. An individual can, of course, have both. Just as an individual with below average intelligence will have conflicts like everyone else, so too will an individual with "below average" developmental levels of one or another tool of ego function have conflicts; all that is affected are the components of the conflict, from the side of the ego. Defects become part of self-definition, become one basis for fantasy development, and thus become involved in conflict. And defects affect the outcome of conflict, bearing on the tools for experiencing and for coping that the person brings to conflict. But what is being emphasized here is that early experiences (with aggressive or libidinal urges and their successful or failed culmination, with object relational needs and their satisfaction or nonsatisfaction)—such early experiences—leave residues, and some of these residues can be aptly described as ego defects. Stating this should make the converse clear: that conflict as we ordinarily think of it, higher-order conflict, requires that basic developmental achievements in the establishment of self and other, in the patterning, directedness, and fantasy elaboration of urge, and in the development of a defense repertoire have all taken place.

In summary, what I have been trying to do in this section is to detail a set of overlapping features of the functioning of every individual that get constructed in the course of early development and, however constructed, once in place have profound consequence for subsequent adaptive/defensive functioning in relation to later psychological demands. I believe that signifi-cant beginnings in each of these areas take place very early on and so can be looked at as preoedipal (in the sense of earlier than the oedipal phase) but here in the domain of the ego psychology. In very concrete ways, however, features such as frustration tolerance, sublimation potential, the attitude to-ward one's own impulses, concern for the object, the development of signal anxiety, and the patterning of libidinal need can be seen as tools, as re-sources (or defective resources in the instance of faulty development), that have consequences for oedipal outcome. Since everyone goes through the storms of oedipal conflict, factors such as these may usefully be seen as among those that help us understand differential outcome. But, beyond this, serious faults in any of these areas can become central focuses of the clinical work in themselves. I have recently come across patients where the regula-tion of tention states, or the attitude toward the urge experience, or repeated negative experiences with mother leading to failed trust and object con-stancy became the center of the work. In each, it proved invaluable to come back again and again to description of these "defects," to attempts at recon-struction of their origins, and to appropriate modifications in technique in order to permit some degree of mastery.

CLINICAL ILLUSTRATIONS

Before giving illustrative clinical material, I should like to comment on a few general points regarding technique as it applies in the area of ego defect. I start with the assumption that some readers will not follow me into my basic premise—that there is, in the instances I will cite, an ego defect; and that others will in any event be cautious on the question of variation in tech-nique. Earlier efforts in this direction are given in my earlier work (Pine, 1985). But let me say, overall, that my own personal leaning (as I have come to be aware of it in my analytic work) is *not* toward a presumption of defect in those patients with whom I decide to work in analysis. I do not think the analytic patient is the main person in whom such defects are seen. But, in the course of an analysis (or so it now seems to me), we may nonetheless come across something that can usefully be understood in such terms. Balint (1968) points out, with regard to certain forms of early disturbance, that patients feel them "to be a fault—not a complex, not a conflict, not a situation" (p. 21). The term *defect* is exactly the same, and makes sense to patients in exactly the same way. Stanley Coen (1986) shows how common the *sense* of defect is—though I do not mean to equate the sense of defect with defect itself.

My own experiences with these problems have come during analyses wherein I was working, in my accustomed way, with the interpretation of conflict as I heard it in the transference, the outside life, and the life history. Ordinarily, this had gone on for some time, at least months and at times a year or years into the analysis. But in each instance, I began after a while to become aware that something felt not quite right. It might be that change in a particular area was even more difficult than it is ordinarily; or that the patient felt in some way not acknowledged or in some way wounded by my interventions; or that the patient said that he or she could not use insight because "something is wrong with me." In the several cases where I became aware of this, my explicit recognition of what I here call an ego defect (but which, of course, in the work I referred to in person-specific ways) produced in the patient a feeling of being understood. I think of instances involving my recognition that the patient seemed unable to bind anxiety and/or depression, or seemed unable to control, or believe he or she could reliably control, certain impulses toward action, or that the patient felt overwhelmed and overstimulated by what seemed to me (not to the patient) to be relatively small and benign interventions. In these instances, when the patient felt newly understood—and usually made this quite clear, with visible relaxation—it led to a further development of the analytic work. But it did not cancel or lead to an end of the conflict-related work that had gone before. Though discovering (recognizing, believing in) the presence of some defect in stimulus tolerance, delay, or object constancy, for example, our work in relation to conflict did not cease. In fact, feeling understood, the patient could generally work more cooperatively and comfortably with the conflictual derivatives as well as participating in the reconstruction of the source of and workings of the defect. So my view remains: it is not a question of defect versus conflict but a question of whether, given a defect component, additional or altered technical procedures may have a place. My sense, further, is that such analytic work is not correctly seen as a preparatory phase to the "analysis proper" that produces an "ordinary neurotic" patient who can then be worked with without parameters. But rather, as we build such things as the capacity to bear tension, to own experience, to retain an inner image of the object, we have basically the same patient we worked with at the start but one who can now be talked to (with less pressing concern for those defects) about the things one ordinarily talks about (interprets) in an analysis—conflict and repetition.

"Is this, then, psychoanalysis?" one might ask. "Or is it psychotherapy?" It is certainly something analysts do, or struggle with. Not all may resolve it as I do; but an engagement with phenomena that at least might be thought of as ego defects, and that are struggled with in the work, occurs during many an analysis. To me, it is an analysis. Patient and analyst are working at it. It does not cease being an analysis merely because some small piece of it occurs in relation to something that is viewed as an ego defect.

Or, in the presence of an ego defect, the question can be asked, "Is the patient analyzable?" I would rather rephrase that to "Is an analysis possible?" And I would often answer yes. But it is not only the patient who must work at it, but the analyst too—with possible modifications of tone, of dosage or titration (Grunes, 1984), and of the holding environment more generally. Also, the kinds of phenomena (such as defects) that are named, recognized, and explored will also be expanded.

Psychoanalysis aspires to achieve structural change in the patient through a process that uses interpretation to reach insight. Expanded cognition, made affectively immediate by seeing phenomena in the transference, and made powerful because insight occurs in a relationship to an analyst who really matters to the patient, is the vehicle for such structural change. But in some sense analysis has arrogated to itself a status as the only treatment that produces such structural change. First of all, that is hardly an empirical generalization; it is an assertion based on some reasonable thinking, some experiences in psychoanalysis, and some attitudes about other forms of treatment—but it is no more than that. I would like to ask, more specifically, might "structural change" not also depend on which "structures" need changing? If we are dealing with failures in object constancy, tension maintenance, or the capacity for delay, might some additional "holding" or "empathic" or individually tailored procedures be the relevant ones for effecting change in that subset of the work? It is at least worth thinking about.

Fleming (1975), in reporting an analysis of a patient with a defect in object constancy, raises similar questions. She writes:

Is it possible that the "alliance" in the therapeutic situation repeats the ego operations that we assume in the establishment of object constancy? Is it also possible that, once the reciprocal relationship is in operation, the terms we use, such as "development of an observing ego," actually refer to the beginnings of a new self image, as well as an "introjection" of an image of the analyst? Is it possible that the structural changes we hope for from the psychoanalytic experience can be facilitated by responses from the analyst other than interpretation in the usual sense of the term? My experiences in trying to understand the clinical phenomena that commonly appear in the course of psychoanalytic therapy have led me more and more insistently in this direction. No adult patient is really a baby, and an analyst is not his parent. Nevertheless, the object need in many adults reproduces in many ways the functional relationship between mother and child—the diatrophic feeling without which the analytic process meets with difficulty. (pp. 748–749)

Fleming illustrates those other-than-interpretive interventions, in her attempt to bring about structural change in an ego defect, in a case that I shall summarize and discuss later in this chapter.

Let me begin with two clinical examples with which I have direct familiarity—one a patient of my own and the other a patient whom I learned about through consultation—and then give two additional examples from the literature.

A Problem in Control of Impulse

A thirty-year-old black female account executive at a brokerage house entered analysis (after previous experiences in psychotherapy) when her new financial position finally permitted her to do so. Both of her parents were social workers, and the idea of psychoanalysis was a familiar one in her home. Ms. K, as I shall call her, had long been troubled by characterological problems centering on inhibition and self-denigration in her personal and sexual relationships. The inhibitions did not seem to affect her work life, however, where she was quite successful and apparently reasonably forceful, though she tended to be somewhat emotionally isolated in work relationships.

The patient was very committed to the analysis, rapidly developed a strong transference which put the analysis emotionally at the center of her life, and brought in considerable material which led to work broadly linked to the character problems that had led her into analysis in the first place.

From early on in the work, and massively intensifying as the work proceeded and the transference relationship intensified, this ordinarily inhibited woman began to reveal a fear that she would be unable to prevent herself from actually approaching the analyst sexually. She was aware of this as an impulse, not just as a thought, and often felt a powerful combination of temptation, shame, and fear of rejection as the impulse mounted. It is this specific feature, which I ultimately came to think of as a circumscribed ego defect, that I wish to focus upon.

Over the course of the first three years or so of the analysis, this impulse of the patient's appeared in the work in innumerable ways, and a variety of interpretations were offered. The interpretations proved productive, in that they contributed to the opening up of considerable amounts of new material about the past, some of which I shall summarize momentarily; the patient also worked well, both associatively and in making use of interpretations, in relation to the various contexts in which this impulse was aroused. One of the central features was her idea that I expected her, as a black woman, to be out of control; at the times when she could experience that as coming from me (that is, from the outside), she could avoid the experience of intrapsychic conflict with her own middle-class, rather moralistic values. But for all of what seemed like good work, and in the context of the patient's being able to make use of insight to alter her life and modes of functioning in other areas, there was essentially no diminution of the urge toward me or the fear of its getting out of control. Quite the reverse; as already stated, it intensified as the transference deepened. It was not always present; but it became a familiar recurrent experience.

Although the patient never in fact acted on this impulse in any clearly manifest way, her fear of acting came to seem not unwarranted. Though it had not been known at the outset, it was learned that each of the patient's parents had been inappropriately sexual with her repeatedly. Her mother, while never actually sexually abusing her, was very physical with her, with much touching until relatively late in the patient's development; and her father, while not physical with her in the same way, drew her into enacted family intrigues, "trysts," and rivalries. Both of these were titillating and confusing to Ms. K growing up, though in ways that she was fairly inarticulate about until the analysis. But even more important, it also emerged that Ms. K had precipitously acted on impulse in the past, in situations of some risk. And additionally, as the impulses toward the analyst grew (and the patient was distressed by this—feeling she would be rejected and then abandoned, or worse, accepted and then find she had lost her analyst as analyst), she began to feel the urge to act outside the analysis, again in potentially self-injurious ways. Impulse control clearly was an issue.

I had no strategy for dealing with what I came to see as a circumscribed but recurrent defect in impulse control. I understood it to be based both on early passive experiences and on identifications with the (sexual) aggressions of her parents as well as on an experienced intensity of need (wish) in the setting of occasional defense failure. But I did respond in ways additional to interpretation. In retrospect, I can see that the following took place, in three steps, and had the effect of stabilizing the patient's control capacity and reducing the fear of loss of control.

The first step was initiated by me. That is, at times when the patient's impulse arose (but also at "cooler" times—see Pine, 1985) "educationally" toned reconstructions were offered regarding the inappropriate parental behaviors and their effect on her as a child. Over time, this permitted an increase in her anger at them specifically in relation to those behaviors, eased her guilt, and allowed her at least to think more easily about her action tendencies.

Sometime thereafter, I noted that the patient started bringing in detailed sexual fantasies about me. But something was different. The quality was now one of enjoying the fantasies rather than being fearful of acting upon them. Much of the time I chose not to say anything about the fantasies themselves—or rather, nothing interpretive. (At earlier stages, as noted, considerable interpretative work had been done.) I saw the patient's pleasurable fantasizing activity as a form of play with ideas, and potentially (I thought) as a step toward self-control. After a while I commented on the fantasizing activity itself, noting that the patient seemed to be feeling safer with her ideas. The fantasizing activity went on for a few months, appearing frequently in sessions, and then faded out.

Somewhat later, the patient began to bring in something else which, in retrospect, I see as a third step in working through the circumscribed impulse control problem. She began to engage in various quite toned down "sexual seduction" enactments. On a number of occasions she paused and looked me up and down (fleetingly) before getting on the couch. Before, and again after, a vacation, she reached out and grabbed for my hand in a handshake—holding it just a moment too long. One Christmas she sent a card that was just a bit too affectionate. In each instance, I suggested to Ms. K that these were forms of safe action to prove to herself that she wouldn't *really* get out of hand, indeed that she *could* act in reserved ways. I described this but in no way interfered with these small actions.

Following those three steps (explanatory reconstruction, play with fantasy, benign enactments), the patient's action tendencies subsided. A fourth element of the patient-analyst interaction may also have played a significant role (Schulman, 1988). I participated with the patient in a particular way, that is, by demonstrating by my behaviour that I could maintain control (unlike the parents of childhood), and thus provided an example that the patient could internalize. After all of this, the patient's fear of losing control essentially disappeared *as a fear*, although it periodically, thereafter, came in as something she would talk about.

I give this brief example (from what in innumerable other ways was just an ordinary analysis) to illustrate a phenomenon that I came to view as an ego defect. I modified technique in small and specific ways in a manner that (I now judge, after the fact) to have been quite useful. Clearly the problem brought by the patient can be conceptualized in other ways as well. We do not have the kind of hard data that permit of decisive proofs.

A *Problem in the Functional Use of Speech*

Mr. L was forty-six years of age when he entered treatment.* He was married and had two teenage children. The immediate precipitant to his seeking treatment was a coronary suffered by a close friend of his which raised his anxiety greatly about his own health. He had long been plagued by hypochondriacal complaints, and the additional anxiety and flood of physical symptoms following his friend's coronary finally spurred him to seek the psychological treatment that his physician had been urging on him for years.

He was also a very quiet man. This, indeed, was the most striking thing about him from the time of the first consultation. He did not give this as one of his complaints, although he did describe less than fully gratifying relation-

---

*I wish to thank Ina Beld, Ph.D., who consulted with me on this work, for allowing me to use the material here. Not having treated this patient myself, I will present a somewhat abbreviated summary.

ships with his wife and children (and others), which could readily be seen to flow from his extreme reticence to speak. In spite of the rather severe inhibition of expressiveness, he seemed a basically intact man and handled his work life and home life reasonably well. He had made a significant adaptation to his quietness. He was a librarian and lived in, as he described it, "a quiet world." By this point in his life, his family did not expect much by way of conversation from him and, though affectionate toward him, they often left him to his reading when they were at home together. What I shall describe as an ego defect here is a soft one—functional rather than structural. Mr. L certainly *could* speak; he had language. The developmental failure, as I conceive of it, was in the failure of speech to achieve a functional role in self-expression and in relating. The body (hypochondriasis) remained a major vehicle for "speech." This view of the patient's silence evolved only slowly during the treatment and was not really given any conceptual label. But the therapist came to believe that such a view of it was productive in the work and enabled the patient gradually to come to experience speech as a part of himself and a part of relatedness. He began to take functional control of it.

From the start of the work, and continuing for a few years into the treatment, the patient was very silent, though not absolutely silent, in the sessions. Speech did not seem to come naturally to him as a means of communication. Gradually it was learned that his family home had been very silent. His depressed father, as he recalls it, rarely said a word. The father had worked in a rather isolated and undemanding position where his silence created no problem, and in the home he simply kept to himself. When the patient tried to speak with his mother, he discovered her to be so preoccupied with keeping the family going (in the face of the father's depression) that she was nonresponsive as well. Mr. L felt unheard. His words seemed to go right through his father; with his mother, unless his words managed to touch on her preoccupation of the moment, they were brushed aside. Mr. L as a child came to feel his words, his inner reality, had no place. All seemed silent to the patient, and he gradually became more and more silent himself.

All of this emerged only very slowly over the course of the treatment. In the sessions, the therapist sat through many long silences with the patient. At times, the therapist felt that the patient was doing in the session what had been done to him—treating the other with silence. At other times it felt as though, in a slight variation of this, he was re-creating the mood of the parent-child relationship—relating through silence. Interventions directed at the resistive aspects of the silence generally went nowhere; the patient simply felt not understood. Silence was his world; it was what he needed to bring to his therapist. It was some years into the therapy before the patient began to make clear that he felt the therapy was his own; it belonged to him and was for him. It was where he could bring his reality, which was silence. As this was conveyed by the patient, he also began to speak more, now using words as well as silence to make himself known to his therapist. At one point around this time he made an explicit statement to his family at the dinner table one evening: "I want to talk more; I want to get more involved with you." This sense in the patient of the therapy being "my own" was seen as a reversal (in the treatment) of the early feeling at home that his reality did not count; there he had no "my own." His father tuned him out; his mother could hear only in terms of her reality. Slowly, speech came to be "my own" also.

Mr. L had a favorite activity. He liked to take long solo hikes on weekend mornings. On them, he was acutely conscious of being silent and alone. He would think of himself as alone in the world with no one even knowing what his voice sounded like. There was little affect connected with this. But at the time when he began speaking more, something changed on his weekend walks. He noticed that emotion entered into his thoughts, emotion in the form of anger. That is, the thought that no one even knew what his voice sounded like was now experienced as an angry, deprived thought for the first time. He felt like screaming it out so that people would indeed know what he sounded like. (In relation to this, let me note that it had often seemed that one defensive aspect of his not speaking had to do with his rage; not speaking was a way to keep the rage silent.)

As noted at the outset, it seemed reasonable to see his not speaking as having a component of ego defect, and useful technically to have done so. It seemed reasonable for two reasons: (1) The extent of bodily symptomatology at the outset (which gradually declined) suggests the possibility that words never sufficiently came to replace the body as a means of expression. Tension of all kinds was still discharged or bound through bodily sensations or bodily fears and fantasies. Words had not fully moved into their potential place in the experiencing, labeling, and communicating of inner life. (2) The silence of his childhood home, and the absence of appropriate response to those communications that he did make, provided only negative feedback for the use of words and no identification models for words as vehicles of communication. The defect is not in speech per se, but in its functional use. Much of speech development occurs in the ambiance of the mother-child interaction (Mahler et al., 1975), which had been lacking in Mr. L's case.

The technical implications that flowed from this stance on the therapist's part have already been alluded to. First and foremost, silence was not considered in this patient to be (primarily) a sign of resistance (though it certainly sometimes had that function as well). Quite the reverse in fact, it was seen as the way he brought vital parts of himself into the treatment; silence was part of him to the core. Interpretations of the silence as a means of avoiding communicating something *else* (rather than as a way of communicating how silence itself was his life), would often have been quite out of touch with him—again substituting another's reality for his own. It would have been (again, in general, not always) unempathic, badgering, wounding. For the therapist to sit through the silences as was done seemed not to repeat the childhood experience, because the patient experienced the therapist as listening, ready, even eager, to speak. And silence itself could be spoken of ("what is the silence like for you?" "is the silence familiar?" "what is your relation to me like during the silence?").

Progress was slow. But speech gradually became something that the patient possessed and used.

The other two cases that I shall present are from the published literature. The first (Fleming, 1975) I shall simply summarize and highlight. The second, Berta Bornstein's (1949) well-known analysis of "Frankie," I shall reconceptualize in terms of ego defect.

A *Problem in Object Constancy*

Fleming (1975) reports on the analysis of an adult man who had had in childhood a severe disruption of his relationship to his mother from the age of four to nine years. Fleming brought to this analysis a history of prior study of early object loss and its impact, as well as an interest in Mahler's concepts regarding the separation-individuation process. The patient brought to the analysis, as Fleming came to understand it, two defects: (1) a relative weakness in the capacity for object constancy—that is, in the capacity to evoke an image of a significant but absent object and to use that image as an internal aid in the regulation of need tension; and (2) "a poorly defined self-image with low self-esteem that needed reinforcement from an external object" (p. 751). The conceptual orientation that the analyst drew upon during the course of this analysis included two points paralleling the patient's defects. First, that object constancy does not develop in a once-and-for-all way in early childhood but that it can suffer later disruptions and that it requires later appropriate inputs. And second, that responses from a significant object, and from the internalized representation of the object, contribute to more adequate self-differentiation and self-esteem—two of the things that were defective in this patient. Overall her argument is based on the idea that any individual has ongoing (as well as early) object needs in addition to drive needs. I shall summarize and discuss this case by quoting from Fleming, in steps, and adding commentary at each step. All page numbers are from Fleming (1975):

> I want to describe and discuss the case of Frank, a man of 32, who presented early in his analysis an extreme reaction to weekend separations. He was an intelligent, competent, financially-successful businessman who suffered from deep-seated feelings of loneliness and inadequacy in his social relationships. . . . The patient's history revealed a very close relationship with his mother during his first four years and I assumed that there had been a constructive symbiotic relationship and an establishment of object constancy. At the age of four, however, his mother was suddenly hospitalized with a chronic illness and he was separated from both mother and father for the next five years, during which he lived with his maternal grandparents. The little boy experienced moments of utter loneliness and despair, wondering if his mother was still alive and feeling that, if he thought about her hard enough, she would not die but would some day return to him. (p. 751)

I would like to highlight two points here. First, though it was Fleming's intent to focus on those small technical variations that were geared to the patient's particular ego defects, it seems implied in the description of him as "an intelligent, competent, financially-successful businessman" that much of the analysis was likely to have been organized around interpretation of conflict as seen in the transference, as in any other analysis; these are not either-or matters of technique. Fleming herself indicates as much at moments in her presentation of the work itself, but it is clearly not her main focus in this paper. My own experience amply demonstrates that work with ego defects does not preclude the carrying out of an otherwise ordinary analysis; it is, in fact, all part of one analysis.

The second point I want to make arises from the fact of a separation at age four, with the presumption of a good mother-child relationship prior to that. Recall that in chapter 9 I suggested that so-called preoedipal pathology may not be preoedipal at all. My main intent there was to suggest that such pathology could be better described in terms of what it *is* rather than what it *comes before* or is *not*. But I suggested, additionally, that once we break out of the conceptual stereotype carried by the term *preoedipal*, we may discover that there are aspects of such other-than-oedipal pathology that are not necessarily formed very early on. I saw the analysis of Mr. E in part in those terms. Here Fleming suggests something similar—particularly when we set the patient's age four in the context of Fleming's earlier theoretical discussion of the *ongoing* aspects of the formation and maintenance of object constancy.

Continuing with the case report,

The analysis began with . . . [a] strong reluctance to become involved. My diagnosis indicated conflict over regressive pulls toward primitive object needs and a poorly defined self-image with low self-esteem that needed reinforcement from an external object. Past experience in such situations influenced me to go slowly, but to encourage him to face his fears and to listen to the fantasies he had when he was alone and felt threatened. He described it as "falling apart" or "not knowing where my head is." At first, my support for his effort to associate in my absence was intuitive, but, as time went on, I realized that it was a response from me that facilitated his ability to evoke an image of me during periods of separation. Subsequent events seemed to validate that formulation. (pp. 751–752)

Here we see the first reported technical variation keyed to the failing in object constancy—association outside of the analytic hour that evokes the memory of the absent analyst. Piaget (1937) has shown that, prior to the development of full object permanence, there is a stage when the infant will continue a search for the now-missing object if he or she has already begun an action sequence in relation to it before it is removed from sight. Action thus facilitates the carrying of memory, before the memory is fully carried independently. The "action" that helped achieve this for Fleming's patient was *associating*.

What I shall describe does not indicate that either the symbiotic relationship with his mother or the earliest establishment of object constancy was historically abnormal. It does indicate that a normal separation-individuation phase may have begun, but that the "hatching out" process was not completed. . . . The actual return [of the mother when the patient was nine] contributed to the complex conflict because, of course, the changes in both mother and son prevented a realistic reenactment of the preseparation situation, a fact that intensified his ambivalence and made the agony of waiting seem to be all for nothing. (p. 752)

So we see here a progressive development of the failure in object constancy. Conflict, "ambivalence," has its role. So too does the failure of the new reality upon mother's return, when all has changed. But the net effect (as seen in the adult patient) is the inability to hold on to the absent other and to use that inner sense of the other in self-regulating ways.

The patient's ability to verbalize what he was experiencing and to make use of my responses made it possible for both of us to work through a series of steps in the development of mental representations that played a part in building a more individuated sense of self and sense of other than he had had before analysis. [Fleming goes on to describe his fear and experience on weekends that the analyst, like mother, would "go poof! and disappear." After a while he recalled (as a child) trying to picture his mother's face and how, after he visited her once in the hospital, it became easier to think of her in her hospital room lying in bed.] In other words, he was using his capacity to evoke an image of a needed object, but he also needed to know where she was. Fraiberg (1969) comments on the advance in organization of a mental representation when the child can call his mother, knowing she must be someplace. [As the patient struggled with the "go poof!" experience, Fleming worked with the idea of spatial localization. After the patient once said that he knew she was gone but would be back on Monday, and added "only I don't know where you are," Fleming] asked if he had thought about where I might be or of calling me. His reply was, "No, I couldn't think about that." [But then he realized he was not as helpless today as he had been as a child, and soon thereafter he came in on a Monday and reported:] "I felt you were gone, but now I know where you are. I found the building you live in and I can picture you there." The next advance in the mastery of separation anxiety was indicated when the patient reported he did not feel so out of touch ever since he could imagine where I was and also imagine my being with someone else. Conjuring up that image produced discomfort, however, because it made him jealous. [And this led to recall of his imagining that his mother enjoyed being with the doctors in the hospital.] (pp. 752–754)

Here we see a second technical modification, Fleming's question whether he had thought about where she was, or of calling her, on a weekend. The patient used that suggestion in his own way, to locate her building, which served as an aid in picturing her whereabouts (and her continued existence). It is of interest to consider that Fraiberg, whom Fleming refers to, may have been particularly attuned to the issue of knowing where the mother is because of her work with blind infants, for whom this is a particularly difficult problem. And Schulman (1988) points out, as in the case of Mr. K where the analyst demonstrated self-control, that again the analyst's participation with the patient in a particular way may have had a significant effect: here, in demonstrating that *she* could be concerned about (and therefore be thinking about) *him* over the weekend. As a last brief comment on the quoted text, the patient's reference to his jealousy is a reminder that issues of conflict, of oedipal wishes, need not be absent merely because a defect in object constancy is present.

Let me give one more of Fleming's technical modifications, and then close with some of her general remarks:

In the psychoanalytic situation, messages are usually communicated by means of the voice. . . . Some patients seem to need visual contact as well. This was borne out in a pattern of behavior that began accidentally with Frank. At the end of the analytic hour, he would sit for a minute on the edge of the couch looking me in the eye. Intuitively at first, I returned his gaze and made a comment or two. Occasionally this exchange lasted for a couple of minutes. When the patient talked of feeling more defined and intact, I began to realize it had the significance that Southwood (1973) and Winnicott(1967) assign to looking into someone's face. He said, "I feel differently about myself . . . I'm responsible for me and can make choices in terms of my own needs. I don't have to fill someone else's space in order not to feel alone and empty." Later still, in the analysis, Frank reported the good feeling associated with these moments and how glad he was I did not interpret what was happening at the time [pp. 754–755]. [This whole exchange seemed linked to an earlier comment of Frank's: "I need you to be with me to know how I feel about myself" (p. 754). Fleming goes on to discuss this as follows:] This patient and I were able to observe phenomena relevant to concepts of object constancy and the symbiosis pertinent to a working alliance, but we could also see the way in which object responses were an important component of experiences which structured a self-image with a sense of positive self-esteem. An effective object constancy was reconstituted in the analytic situation, but there was additional structure building. The development of a working alliance with an object whose internalized image participated in the structuring of a protective evocative memory served as a foundation of security from which self-differentiation and the organization of a self-image developed with a greater sense of self and feeling of self-confidence and self-value than had ever been present before. The constant feeling of inadequacy and vulnerability to external involvements had kept the patient in a state of apprehension about being abandoned, both for inadequacy (sometimes real and sometimes not) and for "being bad." The transference elements in this latter fear were reinforced by the patient's anger and subsequently hostile, aggressive reactions to frustration of his self-esteem needs. (pp. 756–757)

So, once again with the transformations of anger in his "being bad," conflict is present and is worked with. But Fleming's main point is that the face-to-face contact, as the patient sat on the edge of the couch, not only played a further role in the solidification of the internal image of the analyst, but that that image itself, and the patient's ability to carry it inside, is boundary forming (differentiating) and esteem building for this patient.

What we have here, then, is an attempt—created often spontaneously during the treatment—to respond to the patient's defect in object constancy and related capacities, and to do this with small technical modifications in the context of the overall analysis. I emphasize the spontaneity. That is, Fleming, for example, used an act of the patient's (sitting on the couch after a session and looking at her before leaving) to further the work on failed object constancy. She did not bring in a strategy and set of techniques, but responded to the patient's associative (and action) offerings—as one does in any analysis. My work with Mr. K was exactly the same.

I shall close this case with a final quotation from Fleming's paper.

> My experience with adults in an arrested state of development as the result of a death of a needed object in childhood points towards analysis as the treatment of choice. The psychoanalytic situation through its structure and consistency provides security for both patient and analyst, and if the analyst conceives the psychoanalytic process to be comparable to the developmental process, especially in the area of retracking derailed self-object relations, psychoanalytic therapy can be most valuable. (p. 756)

A Problem in Containing Anxiety

The last case I shall discuss is the analysis of "Frankie" presented by Bornstein (1949). This presentation is well known to child analysts and has long been read in child-analytic seminars because Bornstein, a highly esteemed clinician, described not only the analytic work in rich detail but her reasoning process along the way (the choices she made at each step and why). She was sensitive to this child's severe anxiety, and made clear how her timing and tact decisions in the course of the analysis were responsive to it. Still, Bornstein was limited by the concepts and assumptions available to her at the time. She worked with Frankie with the guiding ideas one would use with a neurotic child, albeit one whose severe anxiety required special adaptations. I believe that, today, one would much more readily think in terms of more severe disturbance, and the course of the reported analysis itself demonstrates the more severe pathology. The child responded to the interpretations of each period of the analytic work with the disappearance of one symptom but the creation of another; intrapsychic life tended to remain in major flux, or even to worsen, over the course of the work. Late in the analysis, the emergence of fantasies of omnipotence, of such force and pervasiveness that they disrupted home life and threatened the analysis, led to an actual threat of hospitalization. Only thereafter was there a rapid reduction in the fantasies of omnipotence and a surprisingly rapid (and somewhat unconvincing) move toward a termination phase.

I shall reconceptualize this case in one core way: to suggest that a deep-seated defect in the capacity to bind tension/anxiety underlay the proliferating symptom production. This defect was already evident in (or had its origins in) inconsolable nighttime crying in the first half year of life, and the high anxiety level was evident at times throughout the analysis. The question will be raised whether in this context some other noninterpretive interventions designed to reduce the overall anxiety level might productively have accompanied, or preceded the interpretive work.

I shall try to make my presentation of this case sufficiently self-contained to allow for comprehension; but the reader's understanding would certainly be enhanced by a full familiarity with Bornstein's initial report. I trust many are familiar with the case and others may want to read it afterward. All quotations are from Bornstein (1949).

Frankie, a 5½ year old boy of superior intelligence who was eager to learn, was brought into analysis because of a severe school phobia. . . . He became panic-stricken if his mother or nurse were out of sight [p. 181]. . . . [The history:] The delivery was normal, the child healthy, yet the very first moment [the mother] held the baby in her arms, she had felt estranged from him. The little boy's crying had given her an uncanny and uneasy feeling. She felt quite different toward her second child, a girl [p. 182]. [There follows some historical material about the mother, explaining why this might be so. Then:] Frankie's first disturbance, his constant screaming and crying as an infant, were incomprehensible to the mother. She was convinced that the child's reactions were caused by unsatisfactory feeding in the hospital. And it is a fact that as soon as the intervals between feeding periods were decreased, the screaming attacks became less violent and less frequent. He was a bottle-fed baby and was described as a greedy eater. Night feeding was continued for an unusually long time and when, at the age of 5½ months, the 2 A.M. feeding was stopped, the child again evidenced his discontent. For several months he continued to scream at this hour. It could not be ascertained whether the baby's crying and screaming spells were unusually violent or whether they seemed so because the parents were oversensitive. As a matter of fact, the parents did not dare to fall asleep because of their anticipation of the baby's screaming. When Frankie was 2, it became especially difficult to put him to bed at night. Regularly, he screamed for an hour before he fell asleep, and also whenever he awoke during the night. A third screaming period occurred at the age of 4½ years and was stopped only after the nurse threatened to punish him. (pp. 182–183)

Already, here, we have a basis for thinking of Frankie in terms of some very early disturbance. The first thing to consider is the presenting problem of "school phobia" itself, something today more often described as "school refusal" to differentiate it from the more focal phobias. And such school refusal seems tied to very early separation difficulties, rather than primarily to the kinds of repressed and displaced fear found in those other phobias (such as of dogs, thunder, and so on). And the second thing to consider is the early inconsolable screaming. Chethik (1984), in his research on borderline children, reports such inconsolable periods, often related to early illness and/or pain that the parents could not relieve. Earlier (Pine, 1986a) I suggested that such early states of "overwhelmedness" might be quite widespread in those who later become borderline (and who seem not unlike Frankie), and I try to show the consequences of such states. And altogether the literature on borderline children (for example, Rosenfeld and Sprince, 1963) notes the failure of such children to develop signal anxiety. Bornstein (1949, p. 182) refers to the mother's aloofness with this child, presumably granting it a causal role. But I am reminded of Leo Kanner's (1942) early view of the "aloof" mother of autistic children. In both cases, we have to consider that the mother's response may be a self-protective one to an inconsolable child.

I would suggest that Frankie had some incapacity to bind tension (as reflected in and/or caused by those early screaming episodes). Whether this was due to some inborn drive pressure, or low thresholds, or failure of the parental object, or illness or pain that increased the stimulus overload, the result was still a severe anxiety proneness. In the light of the array of symptoms that he produced before and during the analysis, and in the light of his continued severe anxiety and rage at times during the treatment, clinical caution, I believe, should lead us to consider at least two supplementary hypotheses beyond the usual one that his symptoms represented compromise formations among the various drive/defense/conscience pressures within him. The first, more modest, hypothesis is that the severe anxiety proneness underlay his tendency to produce new symptoms; thus, he would be seen as having started with a handicap, a general vulnerability that made him less adept at successful solutions and more prone to symptomatic outcomes. The second, additional and stronger, hypothesis is that his symptoms, in addition to being compromise formations, were desperate attempts to bind the severe anxiety—as was his response to interpretations. Taking this into the fabric of the analysis itself, I would suggest the possibility that his receptiveness to interpretations (and it is, after all, only though the interpretations offered by Bornstein that we "understand" his symptoms) did not always attest to their correctness but to his desperate attempt to find a "meaning," an "explanation," for his ever present anxiety. These are not either-or matters. I am not suggesting that the symptom formation was random, outside of psychic determinism. I am suggesting that some early predisposition to anxiety, and the process variable of a receptivity to explanation—to *any* explanation that promised to help bind and explain away the anxiety—may also have been factors in the total situation. I say all of this, of course, with knowledge of Bornstein's full report of the analysis, which I have not summarized yet, including and especially the proliferating symptoms and the ultimate near loss of reality testing, neither of which sounds like the productions of a phobic neurotic child.

Bornstein goes on to describe the onset of the analysis. She felt it needed a preparatory period in which Frankie could come to have a reality conflict. In this conflict his school phobia would come to feel like it deprived him of school, where he would also wish to be; and she then describes how this was accomplished: "To be sure, Frankie was already suffering from an internal conflict as shown by his phobia" (p. 184). While I do not doubt the presence of an internal conflict—indeed, of many—Bornstein here is working with the assumptions available to her at the time. School phobia was a phobia and had to do with unconscious conflict and displacement. Ordinarily this meant drive-defense conflict. Consideration is not explicitly given to the earlier screaming periods, and to those somewhat different kinds of "conflict" involved in early separation difficulties. School phobia is, after all, a re-

fusal to separate from the mother. Bornstein's next point about the onset of
the work is consistent with this:

> His dramatic play during his first session led straight into his conflicts,
> just as in adult analysis the first dream often leads into the core of the
> patient's neurosis. His play revealed at once *the experiences that had
> led to his phobia and thus betrayed the meaning of the symptom* [emphasis added]. [Frankie's mother had given birth to his sister when he
> was 3 years and 3 months of age.] Frankie started his first session by
> building a hospital which was separated into a "lady department," a
> "baby department," and a "men's department." In the lobby, a lonely
> boy of 4 was seated all by himself, on a chair placed in an elevated
> position. (pp. 184–185)

From here, Bornstein goes on to describe the session further, focusing on
the "unfaithfulness" of his mother who went away and gave birth, the boy's
sadness, and his defensive grandiosity (the elevated chair). All of this is certainly to the point but, I believe, is overstated as "the experiences that had
led to his phobia." It seems to omit all the early, presumably predisposing,
periods of screaming for contact and comfort. It is not until toward the end
of the case report, after the threat of hospitalization, that Bornstein substantially introduces the earlier material:

> Nothing in our interpretation [of his unrealistic omnipotent beliefs as a
> wished-for reversal of his early infantile helplessness] caused Frankie
> more despair than the analogy between his temper tantrums when his
> wishes were not fulfilled and the attacks of screaming and fury which
> an infant shows when its hunger is not immediately satisfied. Here we
> touched on what we probably might consider his "primal trauma" in a
> period in which he, hungry for milk and affection, screamed for hours.
> This, as the reader will recall, had happened when night feeding was
> stopped at the age of 5 months. (p. 217)

That this child continued to show faulty anxiety binding, and pathology
beyond the neurotic range, is reflected by various asides Bornstein makes as
she is describing the analytic process. Thus: "If a child is only ready to tolerate what the analyst says without covering his ears, he shows that he is mak-

ing the first step in acknowledging the existence of a problem. . . . Children are in much greater danger of being flooded by instinctual demands" (pp. 198–199). And later: "Here the analyst should have become aware that the sense of urgency which [Frankie] betrayed in his actions indicated an attempt to demonstrate more than a mere theory, namely, a past experience which he could not verbalize. Such emotional urgency appears to us as a clinical indication that we are dealing not with a fantasy but with a reality experience—and furthermore, an experience the impact of which probably came before verbalization was possible" (p. 202). And still later, in a session after he heard about the escape of two criminals and during a period when he was beset by a fear of kidnappers: "His first response . . . was to refuse to see the analyst anymore. The next day, against his will, he was taken to her office by his father. As soon as he saw the analyst, he lost all control, burst into tears, and assaulted her. He made attempts to choke her, and threatened to burn down her country house" (p. 213). The binding of tension was certainly faulty.

For completeness, I will briefly sketch out aspects of the course of this analysis. There is no way that I can adequately summarize this long and rich case report. The first period of the analysis centered on the school phobia. The sadness of the rejected boy emerged, as did the hostility, which also was played out in his symptom. His fears of not finding his way back to his mother were paralleled by his angry wish that she disappear. With the reduction of his hostility to his mother, the school phobia was reduced and the "preoedipal period" (p. 190) of the treatment—the mother-oriented period—passed for a time. Then followed a focus on his insomnia which led to primal scene fantasies and fears, oedipal wishes, castration fears, and anxiety about menstruation. It was during this period that his omnipotent fantasies first emerged: he was God (later he had a television apparatus that allowed him to see anything he wanted). At this point they were understood as serving his sexual curiosity. Before these fantasies reemerged in a different context, considerable work was also done on urine retention (linked to castration and impregnation fantasies) and an elevator phobia (in which all of his conflicts found representations). Fears of being kidnapped and, more basically, of passivity, culminated in his major pathological product: he was the omnipotent "King Boo Boo." It was this that looked like a breakdown in reality testing and produced the threat of hospitalization (the feared separation), and it was only this threat which induced him to give up the fantasy.

And the threat repeats the experience at age four and a half years wherein the threat by his nurse led him to give up nighttime crying. This outcome certainly leaves room for questions in our minds.

It is in the light of this course of the analysis that I raise questions of technique as well as of how best to view this child (that is, the question of defect in the capacity to bind anxiety). One can wonder whether the whole analysis, in spite of Bornstein's explicit attention to tact and timing, was overstimulating at the same time as it gave him some cognitive mastery. One can wonder whether some form of soothing or "holding" interaction, tailor-made to the details of this particular case (as they were created and matched to spontaneous opportunity in Mr. K and in Fleming's patient), might not have been useful in a long preanalytic period, or in combination with the early analytic work. In another domain, for example, Kohut (1972) has suggested that "narcissistic rage" decreases, not by a direct interpretive confrontation of it (which only increases narcissistic humiliation and, hence, again rage), but by a slow development of greater self-esteem, in the context of which the narcissistic rage fades away on its own as the self is less vulnerable. Would Frankie's symptoms have declined, not by a direct interpretive approach, but through some attempt to reach the core (if core it is) problem in binding anxiety? Granted, this may be considered to be "not an analysis," but (a) it may be appropriate for the patient; (b) it may foster later analysis; and (c) it may go hand in hand with analysis, as in my case of Mr. K and in Fleming's (1975) case. Certainly the analysis as it was carried out, by an exceptionally highly regarded clinician working with the then-available conceptual tools, is far from entirely satisfactory in its course and outcome.

SUMMARY

In this chapter, I have tried to present a developmentally and clinically derived concept of ego defect. Such defects reflect developmental failures or aberrations in the construction of core tools of adaptive functioning such as tension maintenance, impulse delay and control, and object constancy. I have tried to suggest that the defect versus conflict dichotomy is not useful. Conflicts may lead to, be represented by, be built upon, or coexist with defects. But the defect formulation, at least as I espouse it here, can lead to technical variations that may be specifically appropriate to such a condition. I have tried to illustrate such work.

More broadly, I intend this chapter, in combination with the previous one, to reflect a more differentiated view of other-than-oedipal pathology than is captured by the wastebasket term *preoedipal pathology*. Early, and perhaps sometimes later, disturbances in respect to drive, ego, object, and self permit formulations in their own terms which can enhance our capacity for greater specificity of clinical formulation and intervention.

CHAPTER 11

Infant Research, the Symbiotic Phase, and Clinical Work: A Case Study of a Concept

AT THE FIRST World Congress of Infant Psychiatry in Portugal in 1980, Erik Erikson and Margaret Mahler were invited to offer closing commentaries on the entire program. Having heard all of the research reports regarding the cognitive capacities of the infant presented at that meeting, and the general view of the competent infant's adaptation and learning, Erikson (1980) began his remarks, in a tone both whimsical and plaintive, by asking: "What ever happened to the oral phase?" I should like to pursue that question for just a moment by way of introduction to my thesis in this chapter. Has the research on infant cognition and differentiated relatedness taught us that there is no oral phase? Certainly not the same oral phase that we saw formerly. Things are far more complex, and we need a redefined conception of a phase, which I will come to later. Has the infant research, then, taught us that early orality is not of great importance and that we can therefore ignore it in clinical work? Certainly not; and the researchers make no such claim.

In the present chapter, and in the light of that same burgeoning infant research literature, I should like to focus on a question parallel to Erikson's: What is happening to the symbiotic phase? I should like to review the critique, explore the referents of the term *symbiosis* in infancy, address its status as a "phase," and attempt to underscore the continued relevance of symbiotic phenomena both in clinical work and in infant experience. I use the term *symbiosis* because it is now the familiar one, but I use it with specific reference to phenomena of merger or undifferentiatedness or boundarylessness. It is a concept that was intended by Mahler et al. (1975) to say something about the infant's experience, and the question is how our conception of that experience has to be modified in the light of the new understanding of infant perceptual and cognitive functioning. But it is a concept that was not, after all, created solely to describe the infant. Rather, it was intended to help us understand the possible origins of normal and pathological phenomena of later life—of childhood, adolescence, and adulthood. Psychoanalysis traditionally seeks to understand the roots of such phenomena by tracing them to earlier and yet earlier manifestations, to a time when they may have been a universal of normal development; hence the question of their presence in the infant is of some import.

What are the phenomena of later life that I am referring to? They are of four broad kinds: (1) panic-ridden experiences of dissolution (loss of boundaries); (2) delusional ideas of merger (which may or may not be accompanied by anxiety—which, in fact, may be blissful); (3) severe anxiety about separateness (in contrast to "oneness"); and (4) longings for merger (without experienced loss of boundaries). Each of these vary over a wide range in intensity, duration, disruptiveness, and specific content. If we are to understand them in terms of their roots in phenomena of earliest infancy, we have to confront the question: are normal infantile experiences of merger irreconcilable with the demonstrated cognitive capacities of the infant? I think not, and I shall argue that point here, drawing on the general theme of this book—different moments in which intrapsychic life is organized differently —to do so.

Some current infant researchers and theorists think otherwise. In recent years, experimental research has forcefully demonstrated the impressive cognitive and relational capacities of the infant (see Stone et al., 1973, for an earlier summary). This has led more than one contributor to the literature (Peterfreund, 1978; Gaensbauer, 1982; Horner, 1985; Stern, 1985) to argue that a symbiotic phase concept is no longer tenable. The argument is straightforward: The idea that an infant is unaware of the mother-infant boundary and experiences himself or herself as merged with or undifferentiated from the mother simply is incompatible with the findings regarding the functioning of the infant's perceptual and memory apparatuses. And further, since there are many early indications of specificity of attachment to the primary caretaker (that is, behavioral specificity in relation to her as compared with others), we have further indication of the infant's differentiated functioning.

These arguments are compelling. I should like to respond to them to preserve what I believe is a fuller picture of infant functioning as well as to preserve some of the explanatory potential for clinical work in that fuller picture. But especially, I respond to these arguments here as a demonstration of what I believe to be the power of a moments and four psychologies approach to both development and clinical work. The fact that relatively sophisticated functioning is present in the ego sphere at some moments says nothing about what may be going on in other spheres at other moments in the infant's day.

SYMBIOTIC PHENOMENA, INFANT RESEARCH, AND CLINICAL WORK

Let me begin with a reference, once again, to the familiar story of the blind men and the elephant. Each touches a different part and hence describes the elephant differently. Each of them is in fact reporting on a piece of experience that happens to be the whole of that individual's experience.

So too with many of our views of the human animal, views of psychoanalysts and infant researchers alike. Thus, Freud looked early on and saw the centrality of sexuality. Winnicott looked and saw intimate mother-infant interactions producing a nascent self. Mahler looked and saw what she called symbiosis; and Kohut, still later, looked and saw phenomena of self from yet another perspective. I believe that each of these individuals saw something that is really there. And it is in our interest to see what each of them saw. They were each able to see the particular things they saw because of aspects of the culture of their time and because of particular aspects of their own individual history. In regard to the culture, it seems clear to us at this distance that in repressive Vienna of the late nineteenth century, phenomena of sexuality were highly likely to be conflictual within the upper-middle-class culture within which Freud worked; and so, phenomena of sexuality stood out for him as he listened to his patient's associations. And the death of Freud and the relative antiauthoritarianism of life in the United States produced a culture within the psychoanalytic world that was more receptive to new, inventive, and relatively iconoclastic views such as those of Mahler, Kohut, and others. An individual tendency is at work as well. It seems not unlikely that the phenomena a theorist writes of play a significant role in his or her own functioning and lead to a high attunement to those phenomena in others. Thus, phenomena of sexuality and conflict were apparently central in Freud's self-analysis, which went on hand in hand with the early development of his views. It is a magnificent achievement for an individual to take his or her own sensitivities and perhaps vulnerabilities and convert them into a creative achievement that offers us all something with which we can work everafter.

So, let us turn again to Erikson's plaintive and whimsical remark, "what ever happened to the oral phase?" Cognitive researchers, at least in the reports of their research, seem not to see any oral phase. I do not mean to suggest that they would all argue against its relevance; it simply is not central for their research aims. They do not "see" it in the part of the infant that they "touch." Freud, on the other hand, "saw" the oral phase, but from the vantage point of the free associations of adult patients (in the context, of course, of his general knowledge of infant behavior). Erikson (1950), on the other hand, saw the oral phase, broadly speaking, in aspects of the infant's *cognitive* functioning itself; that is, he emphasized, for example, how the infant takes in the world with his or her eyes. His intent was to show that what he called the oral *mode* applied not only to the mouth but to the whole passive, receptive stance of the infant—for example, in the passive receptivity of its perceptual apparatuses.

Let me take the example of a symbiotic phase similarly. Mahler (1968) felt that she saw what she referred to as symbiosis in certain psychotic children, and she described a syndrome of symbiotic psychosis of early infancy. Later she looked for the origins and transformations of such symbiotic phenomena in normal children. At the outset she more or less assumed these phenomena were present and undertook to study how the person developed beyond them—a development that went awry (again, as conceptualized by her) in symbiotic psychotic children. Broadly speaking, she came to believe that a sense of boundarylessness—a lack of differentiation from the other—was affectively and cognitively central to the infant in the earliest months of life, perhaps from the second or third month through the fifth or sixth; she argued that the developmental tasks of early infancy included the task of overcoming that lack of differentiation and achieving a sense of an I-you boundary as part of the development of reality testing. I shall not review her research here. But we come full circle back to the original questions: in the light of the findings of the new infancy research, can we still think in terms of early merger phenomena? as a phase? and, if so, in what sense?

My own view is that it all depends on which part of the elephant you are touching. Much of the infant research touches that part of the "elephant" in which the infant is in what Wolff (1959) long ago called states of alert inactivity, and in which cognitive functioning is at its most reality-attuned point. Some of the research relates to other states, of course, but that does not negate the fact that there are always yet other states, and yet other moments, when yet other phenomena may be central—and these, I will argue, include some which contain the possibility of affectively significant merger experiences. Just as an example of variation: on the day on which I was writing this chapter, a patient reported an experience he had had in a half-awake, half-asleep state that very morning. He had a conviction that the exercise bicycle that he rode on most mornings was broken in a particular way (the significance of which we later analyzed). It took several moments after awakening for him to realize fully that the bicycle was not, in fact, broken and that it was time to pull himself out of sleep and onto his bicycle. Those two moments, the half-asleep one and the waking one, gave him two quite different and, within their own terms, equally convincing views of "reality." The infant's experiences of "reality" presumably also vary from moment to moment.

The infant research literature shows us a great deal about the moments in which the child's perceptual/cognitive apparatuses are attuned to external reality, an area of functioning that psychoanalysis has subsumed under the concept ego. The literature shows how these capacities tie the infant in to the relationship to the primary caretaker (Sander, 1977). And Stern (1985) makes a further case for how all of this contributes to the early formation of a self.

I do not question, in principle, these early developments within the domains of ego, object relations, and self. It is precisely my argument in this entire book that phenomena in the domains of each of the four psychologies are present virtually from birth onward and undergo development through-out the life cycle, as discussed in chapter 4. For me the question is not whether these ego, object-relational, and self-formative capacities are pres-ent but whether they exclude the presence of other "capacities"—that is, the capacity to register yet other kinds of experience. Might there not be special experiences of merger as the infant falls into sleep at the mother's breast? Or are we to believe that this cognitively advanced and finely attuned infant registers nothing of psychological importance at those moments?

Stern (1985) writes:

> Recent findings about infants challenge these generally accepted time-tables and sequences [regarding symbiosis and self-other differentia-tion] and are more in accord with the impression of a changed infant, capable of having—in fact, likely to have—an integrated sense of self and of others. These new findings support the view that the infant's first order of business, in creating an interpersonal world, is to form the sense of a core self and core others. (p. 70)

But who is to decide what the infant's "first order of business is"? Might not a great deal of business be going on all at once? Nothing we know about human functioning supports a notion of single-mindedness. How can we conclude that the infant organism, now shown to be vastly more psychologi-cally alert and complex from birth onward, is thus single-minded? And, fur-ther, if the "first order of business in creating an *interpersonal* world is to form the sense of a core self and core others," what of "orders of business" in the intrapsychic world—the world of sensation, fantasy, and unreality? The infant research critics of merger/boundarylessness phenomena are not ex-actly throwing out the baby with the bath water; they are keeping their baby (the reality-attuned baby) and throwing out other people's baby. But this other baby—the baby of merger experience—may not be any less reality at-tuned. She is just recording her own *experiential* reality (as I will attempt to show), a reality that happens not to accord with objective reality as it will later come to be understood.

Stern goes on in the passage just quoted:

The evidence also supports the notion that this task [forming a sense of a core self and other] is largely accomplished during the period between two and seven months. Further, it suggests that the capacity to have merger—or fusion-like—experiences as described in psychoanalysis is secondary to and dependent upon an already existing sense of self and other. The newly suggested timetable pushes the emergence of the self earlier in time dramatically and reverses the sequencing of developmental tasks. First comes the formation of self and other, and only then is the sense of merger-like experiences possible. (p. 70)

This is a reasonable assertion; but it is only that—an assertion. Another assertion is also possible: the emergence of self and other as well as the laying down of vague memory traces of merger experiences are both occurring simultaneously from the beginnings of life. Again I would not oppose the notion of a very early beginning development of self; earlier (Pine, 1982) I published a paper arguing, and hypothetically detailing, that very development. But why the need for either-or thinking? Of course later fantasies of the merger of a differentiated self and other can be formed. The question is, are they built on yet earlier experiences? I believe that a view of the infant in terms of differential organization at different moments—the view underlying the entire four psychologies approach proposed herein—permits a tentative yes answer. At the very least, it prevents a simplistic answer of no.

Given what we are now learning about infant cognition, yet retaining what we have heard from patients about merger experiences, I would propose that the infant has *moments* of the experience of boundarylessness or merger—not an ongoing state of weeks' or months' duration. My prime candidate for such moments of merger are those moments when the infant, in the mother's arms, having sucked vigorously at breast or bottle, progressively calms and falls into sleep as body tonus relaxes and he or she melts into the mother's body. Cognitive functioning is certainly not likely to be at its best during these moments. The reality-attuned cognitive performances of the infant will be mainly during the periods of alert inactivity (Wolff, 1959) which occur sporadically through the day (and for progressively longer time periods through the early months), but not at moments of vigorous sucking, melting into the mother's body, and falling asleep. A sense of boundarylessness can be present; and, conversely, articulated awareness of boundaries (associated with the moments of higher cognitive functioning) will fade. There is clearly no contradiction between the presence of such moments of merger in the postfeeding drowsy state and the presence of more articulated cognition in other states. Whether the moments of falling asleep into the mother's body are the only such moments of merger experience, or whether, for example, moments of intense mutual eye-to-eye gaze or mutually responsive cooing and babbling are also such moments for the infant is in no way critical to the argument I am advancing. What is critical is that there are at least *some* moments of the merger experience.

But these are only the intense moments. The many quiet and sustained background moments when the half-asleep infant is cradled in the mother's arms, sensing her warmth, her smell, her sounds is another prime candidate for subjective merger experience. And perhaps other moments, too, may contribute to such experiences. I have in mind those moments when the infant is being carried in the mother's arms while she is in motion, the infant moving with her body, the two of them in complete synchrony. The infant's day provides many moments when the subjective reality of the infant's experience may be one of merger or boundarylessness.

But this brings us to another possible argument against such notions. Will not the infant's more "realistic" differentiated perceptions of mother-self separateness be the dominant ones? Won't they provide a stable anchor of perception and memory that erases the more "fantastic" merger experiences? Aside from the point that those merger experiences may not be so "fantastic"—that is, they may be the *reality* of experience at some times— there is every reason to believe that the more realistic (in adult terms) differentiated perceptions will not automatically be dominant. They are not reliably dominant in all adults, even when the fact of self-other differentiation is far more strongly established. In fact, if the realistic perceptions were automatically the dominant ones, there would be no need for psychoanalytic or dynamic psychotherapeutic treatments at all. Quite the reverse is the case. Psychoanalysis teaches us how extraordinarily difficult it is (in selected areas of conflict) for objective reality to win out over the reality powered by wish and affect.

And there is a second reason, this time solely from within the domain of infant development, to believe that moments of awareness of separateness do not achieve dominance over moments of the experience of merger (Hegarty, 1989). That is, whatever has thus far been demonstrated about the infant's cognitive capacities, we still have no evidence that the infant has the capacity for a superordinate cognition that compares, contrasts, and/or reconciles divergent cognitive impressions, choosing one over the other.

The impact of affect and wish on realistic perceptions offers a whole other mode of rejoinder (in addition to the "moments" conception) to an argument for the automatic centrality of those cognitive differentiations of which the infant is capable when functioning at his or her highest cognitive level. Thus, in a related sphere, McDevitt (1975) argues that the constancy of the internalized libidinal object is challenged—even after it is attained—under the barrage of the infant's rage. I developed (Pine, 1985) McDevitt's initial argument further as follows:

> Factors in the post eighteen-to-twenty month period must also be taken into account in a comparison of physical object permanence (cf. the work of Piaget, 1937, on the child's achievement of a concept of the permanence of *inanimate* objects) and libidinal object constancy. The libidinal object is subject to extremes of longing and rage, and the representation of that object may be wishfully or defensively distorted or protected (McDevitt, 1975). This is not true of the physical objects Piaget studied—and indeed, if it were, they would be libidinal objects in our sense. Thus we cannot even assume that once permanence of the physical object has been attained, constancy of the libidinal object has also been attained. We can only say that the cognitive potential is there. The presence of intense libidinal and aggressive ties to the object may thus make for *more rapid* but *less fixed* attainment of a permanent cognitive/affective representation of it in all its aspects. (p. 104)

The argument with regard to the wishful and affective challenges to the constancy of the libidinal object applies identically to the challenges to the "attained" differentiation of self and other in the infant.

Jacobson (1983) has applied ideas regarding moment-by-moment variation to the clinical situation, showing how interpretations are variously directed one way or another at different moments. In response to an earlier publication (Pine, 1986b) in which I set forth some of the arguments presented here, Jacobson (1987) wrote to me as follows:

> I have been approaching from a clinical standpoint, along lines which may be of interest to you, some aspects of the same dilemma you ad-

dress in your paper. As you say, there is much at stake clinically, as well as in a broader scientific sense, in how we eventually interpret and utilize the mounting number of observations of previously unpredicted perceptual capacities in neonates and young infants. The dilemma for the psychoanalytic clinician and teacher, of course, is how to keep abreast of these new data, and integrate them into our thinking, without prematurely jettisoning valuable clinical concepts, such as the various symbiotic phenomena. Your differentiation of states of alertness from states of somnolence is most helpful in this regard. We have a variety of indirect means by which we gain access to the older child's and adult's world of somnolence. Free associations, reported dreams, constellations of behavior, empathic resonance with unverbalized ego states, etc., all lead us to the relevant unconscious fantasies. I found helpful your pointing out that much of the current infant observational research leans heavily on observable behaviors during states of arousal and alertness and less on inferred inner affectual experiences of the somnolent state. It strikes me that gaining access to the infant's world of somnolence, to gather data naturalistically, without "waking" the infant to alertness, requires even more patience and ingenuity than it has taken to evolve these techniques for the verbal child and the adult. The severely narcissistic or even schizophrenic patient who might satisfy for many observers the criteria for inferring a merger state with mother, would still in many observable everyday behaviors appear to treat her as a separate individual [and here Jacobson is recognizing the momentary variations, now in the schizophrenic, as I pointed out in respect to the patient and his exercise bicycle or the infant with respect to differentiation and undifferentiation] and would therefore demonstrate apparent self-object differentiation on an adult equivalent of the perceptual tests used in early infant observational research. He looks towards her when she talks, doesn't try to occupy the same chair that she does, etc. And yet he might satisfy us clinically that unconsciously he firmly believes the two of them to be "really" one, sharing thoughts, affects, bloodstream, nervous system, and fate. What we are referring to in these instances as "merger" is, of course, an inferred unconscious fantasy or affective experience of merger, an enduring or repetitive ego state, rather than an intellectual assessment by the patient.

I have thus far in this chapter been developing the idea that, as in the case of the four psychologies, there is moment-to-moment variation in the way experience is organized. I would like now to continue my argument along an additional line—that is, the spread from moments to larger segments of experience, segments that become affectively central and problematic for some developing persons.

MOMENTS, MAGNIFICATION,
AND MOTHERING

Can such brief moments of merger carry the developmental weight that our theories give them? Can they help account for the place of symbiotic phenomena in psychopathology and normal development? To me there is no doubt that they can. There is certainly no direct correlation between the temporal duration of a psychological phenomenon and its degree of impact on development or functioning. The simplest and most vivid example I can adduce is the orgasm. Consider the amount of time spent in orgasm during a week and the degree of its importance to us as functioning adults. Surely the proportional importance far outstrips the proportional time spent!

I have suggested elsewhere (Pine, 1985) that these symbiotic moments are affectively central ones in the infant's day and thus have a developmental significance far beyond what mere duration would predict. Whatever the cognitive capacities of the alert infant at the moments when they are assessed, we might speculate that these affectively significant merger experiences color the infant's inner experience of his or her world for much larger blocks of time. This idea is part of what we have in mind when we speak of early experiences being organized along affective lines (that is, "good experiences" and "bad experiences") rather than conceptual ones (Freud, 1915; Rapaport, 1951; Kernberg, 1976). Later in the infant's development, when the concept of the separateness of self and mother is clearly and more firmly laid down in memory, the momentary experiences of merger may (in the normal case) be less prone to spread to a general sense of boundarylessness.

Not every person, however, represents this normal case. For the infant,

one of the routes by which a giant step is taken from momentariness to lasting significance has to do with the intersect of the phenomena of some particular moment with highly emotionally laden issues of the mother's
functioning. *When the child's moment meets the mother's character or conflicts, a magnification of the moment is likely to take place.* We can imagine
many scenarios (and see Mahler et al., 1970, on mothers' reactions to their
childrens' separation and individuation). Thus, a mother for whom the infant's melting into her body is a vital emotional necessity, who holds, and
cuddles, and conveys her longing at such moments—and who, contrariwise,
is depressed or otherwise unresponsive at other moments—will automatically, by her very response, magnify the psychological significance of those
moments for the infant. Or another mother, who responds with irritability
and/or sadness to the child's moments of individuation (say, a "no" or tod-
dling off on his own) will imbue those moments with conflict and/or loss for
the child, at times pulling certain predisposed children back to less individuated functioning. Such magnification of the significance of moments potentially occurs with respect to all developmental phenomena, and actually
occurs with at least some for every mother-infant pair. For some it is the
merger moments, for others orality, or toilet training, or gender confusion,
or sexual curiosity, or triadic rivalries. What matters in the mother's character and conflicts will come to matter in the child's moments, thus extending
their significance beyond the moment, and will ensure their spread into the
child's character and conflicts. In such ways does a magnification of
momentary experience occur.

After thus bringing in the role of mothering in highlighting merger-
differentiation experiences for particular infants, I should like to return
to Stern's (1985) argument that merger fantasies are *later* developing
phenomena, whereas the period from two to seven months sees the consolidation of a core (differentiated) sense of self and others. I have no
doubt that merger fantasies, like any other fantasies, are progressively
elaborated throughout the life course as cognition becomes more advanced and experiences are recorded in memory. But the role of those
magnifications (of merger/differentiation phenomena) that stem from
psychological issues *in the mother* point to very early origins. For it is
with the helpless and "fragile" baby of the first half year—the baby whose
head needs supporting, who regularly melts into mother's body when he
or she is in her arms—that the mother's own deep-lying merger issues

and fantasies are likely to be activated. And if the mother's conflictual (either avoidant or absorbing) response to the infant's helplessness has a magnifying effect on the infant's experience, it is likely to start doing so at this very early age.*

With this discussion of the way particular moments become emotionally salient for one or another developing infant and child, my focus flows back naturally to the clinical situation. For some individuals, when they arrive in our offices, the phenomena I described earlier are central in their functioning: panics over merger, or over separateness; delusions of merger; longings for "oneness." It is the existence of such clinical phenomena that produces the whole interest in early merger experiences, and some attempt to understand how they become central for some persons—whether longed for, feared, imagined delusionally to be present, or in fact present in some background way (Winnicott, 1958a) where the other is carried inside as a source of contact and comfort. Because such experiences are seen as having their origins in particular moments of infancy, there is nothing here that contradicts the findings of the new infancy research, which focuses on what the infant's experience may be like at *other* moments. But because of the potential affective centrality of the moments of merger, especially when magnified by interaction with the mother's conflictual affective life, they enable us to understand something about the source and power of those later panics and longings regarding differentiation and undifferentiation that, at the very least, we must consider *may* stem from early experiences such as those I have postulated.

CONCLUDING REMARKS

The whole tenor of my discussion requires the redefinition of what we refer to as a phase in development. For, in the present instance, if we are

---

*A parallel age-linked issue regarding affective significance bears on the question of the infant's early capacity for self-other differentiation. It may be, as the new infant research suggests, that the infant is *capable* very early on of such differentiation (at least at moments), but the presence of the eight-month stranger and separation anxiety implies that these capacities first take a problematic affective meaning at that *later* age and that, therefore, the earlier discrimination capacity now has a new functional significance.

left only with moments of merger the idea of a symbiotic phase requires revision. What can be said about the idea of a symbiotic phase? Surely a
phase is more than a collection of such moments. In fact, I think it useful
to define a phase quite differently. I have developed this argument elsewhere (Pine, 1986b), but for the sake of completeness here let me restate
the major points. A child no more spends all his or her time being "symbiotic" in the symbiotic phase than he or she does being "oral" in the oral
phase or "anal" in the anal phase or "oedipal" in the oedipal phase. In all
such phases the child is a multifaceted, cognitively complex being—far
more so than the libidinal phase terminology indicates. Libidinal urge, aggressive urge, exploration and play, self and object experience, developments in ego and superego function are all parts of all such phases. But in
all such phases, the psychological phenomena that give the phase its name
also have an affective centrality that far outweighs considerations of mere
temporal duration.

I have proposed redefining a phase as the period in which the critical formative events in any particular area of development take place, without regard to the momentariness or temporal spread of those events. And these
critical formative events can be organized around affectively central, even if
momentary, phenomena. Thus, returning specifically to the focus of this
chapter, the symbiotic phase is the time of the critical formative effects of
those moments of merger (associated with nursing and falling into sleep
while melting into the mother's body) that take place in the earliest months.
The same would hold true for phases or orality, anality, gender identity formation, or the oedipal constellation. None of these terms refers to a totality
of the child's experience but rather, I suggest, to a time when the critical formative events with respect to each of those phenomena take place. And
these critical formative events are, in each instance, affected by caretaker
interactions in which the emotional issues of the caretaker magnify some
experiences for the infant or child.

It should be recognized that this is quite a different conception of the
symbiotic phase than the one initially presented by Mahler (1972; Mahler et
al., 1975). The findings of the infant research literature certainly have affected this conception. Moments of merger are different from a symbiotic
totality. This presents a different view of what the baby is like in the first half
of the first year. But it is a view that nonetheless, in its preservation of a place
for merger phenomena, permits all the conceptual work necessary to pro-

vide a framework for the understanding of the later tasks of separation and individuation, as well as for the pathology of failures of differentiation, and it does so without contradicting the data of the new infancy research. And it is also a view of the infant that gives space (moments) for all of those phenomena that are the origins of what we later come to think of as the psychologies of drive, ego, object relations, and self.

CHAPTER 12

On the Mutative Factors in Psychoanalytic Treatment

THE LAST QUESTION that I shall address is, what is it in the psychoanalytic process that brings about change? I believe that a four psychologies view can enrich our appreciation of the breadth of such mutative factors. By alerting us to different aspects of mind, they alert us to a wider range of therapeutic happenings. I shall, in what follows, address these in terms of each of the four psychologies first for verbal interventions and insight and then for relational effects of the treatment. This division itself implicitly reflects the various psychologies—for the power of insight is embedded in a theory of the ego, of cognition and learning and affect transformation, and the power of relationships is embedded in both the theory of object relations and the self, the latter seen as taking shape in relation to the other (Spitz, 1957; Mahler, 1972; Kohut, 1977). What follows will be a sample of issues in the psychology of change, meant to illustrate the utility of a view from the position of the four psychologies.

VERBAL INTERVENTIONS

To be effective, a verbal intervention must be in some sense true—that is, it must touch the patient's experience so that he or she can resonate with it. To do this, I believe, requires interpreting at different times within one or another of the varying conceptual frameworks of the several psychologies. Thus, the background of the views I shall present here is provided for by this entire book. In particular, the series of questions in chapter 3, generated by an expanded view of evenly suspended attention, and the broad view of significant areas of development outlined in chapter 4, provide a background for interpreting within the domains of drive, ego, object relations, and/or self, as appropriate.

Regarding the psychology of drive, I am of course in the familiar center of classical psychoanalytic technique and shall be brief. Making the unconscious conscious, and "where id was there shall ego be" (Freud, 1933) have reference to the interpretation of unconscious conflict, powered by conscience, using ineffective or rigid defenses, and operative against unacceptable urges or wishes. The therapist's task is interpretation, with the aim of gradually producing modification of conflict, conscience, and inflexible modes of defense, all permitting reorganization to take place with greater success in the patient's acceptance of thoughts and urges, in conflict resolution, affect tolerance, displacement, and sublimation. Especially when the analytic process is stuck in some way, or on those occasions when complexly interwoven material has come together within the confines of a single hour (see Kris's "good analytic hour," 1956b), the power of interpretation of unconscious conflict—its power to move the process forward—is truly impressive.

In relation to the psychology of internalized object relations, where early experiences are seen to be repeated in part because of the stress associated with them (repetition in efforts at mastery) and in part because of the pleasure associated with them (repetition in efforts at gratification), the therapist's task is, once again, interpretation, with the aim of freeing the patient to meet new experience as *new*, without absorbing it into the old drama of historically based object relations. Transference, which can be understood in terms of the continuing pressure of urges to be expressed and which are played out on the person of the analyst, can equally be conceptualized as the tendency to repeat old internalized object relationships. Here, too, the power of interpretation to bring about a sudden new perspective on what is going on in an analysis (in the transference) or in the patient's life outside, and to move the process forward, is compellingly clear.

In the regions both of drive and of internalized object relations—that is, with respect both to unconscious wishes and to unconsciously compelled repetitions of old object relationships—interpretation brings the power of the patient's cognitive apparatus to bear and permits him or her to see and to change habitual ways. If this were all there were to it, however, analyses would be a lot shorter than they are. Seeing and *believing*, seeing and *remembering*, or seeing and *changing* are clearly not coincident with one another, and the patient's attachment to the old wishes and/or relationships is not easily renounced; and so analysis as we know it, with continual discovery, rediscovery, and working through, is the expectable mode. And I should add, parenthetically, that the fact that this takes place within a powerful relationship is altogether what gives it the chance of being more than just words. It is the immediacy of interpretation in the transference that makes it *real*, and the intensity of the patient-analyst relationship that makes it *matter*.

Still, it is clear that interpretation does not always lead to change. Freud's concepts of "adhesion of libido" (1916) and "resistance of the id" (1926) essentially merely gave recognition to the fact of nonchange—when fact it was—without really clarifying anything. And Eissler's (1953) concept of parameters essentially legitimized what analysts were learning that good technique required—namely, doing different kinds of things at times.

So, with this in mind, and turning to the regions of self and ego pathology, the situation regarding interpretation can be seen to be different. Though lines cannot be sharply drawn and there are no either-ors in this work, still an "interpretation" of a *defect* in ego function or of a *deficiency* in parental input producing a faulty self experience does not in itself lead to a useful "now I see" experience. The relational aspects of the analytic encounter may play an important role here, but I will come to that later. For now, let me stay with aspects of verbal intervention and their impact. What makes interpretation potentially mutative with an unconscious urge or wish and the anxieties and defenses associated with it is that the conflict dates from the childhood era where it might have seemed to make sense (such as the threat of castration for certain wishes) but can be judged differently in light of adult reality. And the mutative potential of interpretation of repetitions of old internalized object relations similarly rests on the presumption that, today, having a life separate from the parents of childhood, the patient can be different. But interpretations that make the patient see, for example, defects in the subjective self experience (low esteem, shaky boundaries, discontinuity) pose the danger of rubbing salt in wounds or of eliminating hope and merely causing pain.

In areas of primary deficiency, verbalization may have a significant mutative potential when it comes in the form of description, explanation, and reconstruction—especially within the overall holding context of the analytic relationship (Modell, 1984). The aim is to help the patient to become familiar with these inner states, to bring them into the sphere of verbalization and shared understanding, and to help understand how they came about in the family history. My experience is that this gradually enables the patient to better bear the pain of such states by becoming familiar with their quality, triggering events, course, and source (though it does not eliminate the pain), which in turn permits bearing (sustaining) them rather than acting upon them. But in other regions of self disturbance, interpretation certainly has a role—and it shades over into what I am calling description or explanation or reconstruction. I have given illustrations of such interpretations in chapter 3.

In relation to the psychology of ego function, much of what we work with in a psychoanalysis with a reasonably intact patient is clinically inseparable from interpretive work on drive and conflict. The whole area of rigid, malfunctional, ineffective, and outdated defense is at the core of such interpretive work and is familiar enough. On the other hand, the area of ego defect—that is, the faulty initial development of basic tools of functioning—requires comment exactly parallel to that of defect in the self experience. Interpretive interventions often produce helplessness, depression, or narcissistic mortification. Yet, as with defects in the self experience, to describe, explain the workings of, and reconstruct the origins of such defects can be a positive step in the treatment that, at the minimum, permits the patient to feel recognized, understood, not alone with the defect, and gradually to come to some terms with it; these are essentially reconstructions, which the patient receives educatively. I have tried to illustrate work with such ego defects in chapter 10.

Let me assert a number of points regarding verbal intervention and change before continuing. (1) Interpretation, bringing consciousness and the power of the cognitive apparatus to bear on inner life, is a powerful mutative factor in psychoanalysis; (2) it is most effective in an intense patient-analyst relationship where every communication from the analyst *matters* to the patient; (3) it is ordinarily most powerful when linked to the transference, where it is most immediate and real; (4) (and this is a more distinctive part of my argument) interpretation is most effective when it is most true (and *true* here means touching the patient's experience so that he or she resonates with what has been said), and this requires working with shifting theoretical models—in our current language, models of drive, ego, object relations, and self; and (5) in areas of defect—notably regarding aspects of the faulty development of self experience or of functional tools of adaptation —interpretation can at times produce painful confirmation without therapeutic impact, though other modes of verbalization—describing, explaining, reconstructing—can produce familiarity, some degree of acceptance, a capacity to bear, and modest change as well.

Until now, in discussing the verbal interventions that the analyst makes, I have been attempting to show how the analyst's behavior can be productively influenced by having conceptions of each of the four psychologies in the back of his or her mind. Schafer (1983), in his emphasis on diverse psychoanalytic narratives, and Jacobson (1938), in his explicit use of structural theory and representational world theory (in an analysis of the psychoanalytic encounter) are recent forebears of this kind of effort—though each in quite different ways.

RELATIONAL ASPECTS OF THE THERAPEUTIC ENCOUNTER

In this section, I use the four psychologies as conceptual tools to analyze a process that simply happens under the special circumstances of a clinical psychoanalysis. Patients use the relationship with us, and experience us, in ways that foster the analysis, support resistance, feel to them like condemnation, punishment, or humiliation on the one hand, or love, praise, and special attention and guidance on the other. Much of this eventually becomes clear and is itself subjected to analysis if all goes well. But after what is conflictful, and in that sense "noisy" and noticeable, enters the analysis and is gradually pared away, there remain other ways in which we are functional in the psychic lives of patients—ways that are relatively conflict free and that contribute to the mutative power of the analytic encounter. I wish to describe some of these now.

To begin, then, from the standpoint of the psychology of drive: the *absence of condemnation* that accompanies the analyst's inquiries, observations, and interpretations with respect to wishes that the patient regards as taboo, can gradually lead to modification of conscience, as Strachey (1934) pointed out long ago. Additionally, the fact that the analyst continually *survives*, in the sense of not being drawn into reciprocal sexual fantasy or behavior and not retaliating with rage or rejection in the face of the patient's rage, provides a model for the patient to follow. The situation is as Winnicott (1963a) described in the infant-mother relationship: the mother who repeatedly survives the infant's destructiveness enables the infant to learn that his or her destructiveness will not destroy, can be safely (gradually) owned, and can be expressed even toward loved ones. The patient in analysis, both through repeated talking of wish and fantasy regarding both sexuality and rage, and through observation of the analyst's matter-of-fact response, learns that "nothing happens"—no action, no seduction, no condemnation, no retaliation. Just survival, going on with life. While, to be sure, at times this leads to disappointment, further provocation, fantasied condemnation, or wished-for action, as analysis of all of these continues, what remains is survival. Life goes on, now with formerly taboo wishes simply owned.

From the standpoint of the psychology of object relations: One core feature of an analysis is its provision of a new, corrective object relationship for the patient, one that can gradually enter into the world of internalized object relations. I do not say this with instructional intent; I am not suggesting that the analyst "should be" this way or that—nice, helpful, or what have you. What I am saying is that the analyst, with his or her sustained attention, concern, noncondemnation, and persistent efforts to understand, *is* different from the internalized parent of childhood. It has long been recognized that the child analyst is a new object and not only a transference object to the child patient; I do not believe this ever fully disappears, even for adult patients (see Loewald, 1960). Yet if the patient steadily experienced the analyst as a new object, something of the necessary storm and stress of the analytic relationship would surely be missing. Rather, what is new and corrective is that the patient can continually rediscover, following analysis of transference distortion and following mutual recovery from the analyst's errors and empathic failures, that the analyst remains basically well intentioned and concerned. Additionally, the work generally moves in that direction over time. If the patient, nearing termination, is unable to view the analyst with reasonably consistent trust, and with a sense that he or she has been able to be helpful and clarifying at least some of the time, surely we would feel that something had not gone well.

A second object-relational component of the analytic encounter with mutative effect is what Loewald (1960) has addressed in his discussion of the disintegrative and integrative experiences of an analysis. The free associative process, and the couch, and the analyst's silence and interpretations continually lead to mini-disintegrative experiences; the analyst's intervention (or, sometimes, mere presence) permits new integrations to occur, and, through these, progressive mastery. But it is precisely the background object relation with the analyst, on the model of the parent-child relation, that permits these integrations to occur.

And now, third, from the standpoint of the psychology of the self—still looking at effects carried by the patient-analyst relationship in itself: Here, of course, Kohut's (1971, 1977) work is most explicit on the subject. Not only does he point out that the patient's experience of feeling "mirrored," empathically understood, by the analyst and/or idealizing the analyst can in part compensate for deficient experiences of the patient's childhood that have contributed to a lack of esteem and well-being in the self experience, but additionally he cautions against interpreting these experiences too early out of the analyst's ultimately countertransferential discomfort that he or she is not being sufficiently "analytic," that is, is allowing the idealization or the patient's pleasure in feeling mirrored. His point is that, while interpretation (or, in my terms earlier—description, explanation, and reconstruction) has a significant place, so too, and especially in deficit states, does *experiencing*.

And beyond these specific narcissistic transferences, as Kohut called them earlier on (1971), it is my impression that all patients take something of that sort from the analytic encounter. Though it is often slow in coming (because so much of the therapeutic dialogue pertains to the patient's self-perceived "badness") generally the patient slowly comes to feel valued by the therapist—valued enough to be worked with in the face of perceived badness and valued enough for the analyst to be reliably there, attentive, and working in sessions day in and day out, year in and year out. Certainly that has an effect at least in small ways on self-esteem.

In another area that I have subsumed under issues of self—the area of self-other boundary formation—I have also been impressed by the effect of the direct experiential aspect of the treatment situation. Ms. A (reported in chapter 7) put that into words frequently. The sense of "perfect communion" between us was both like that between herself and her mother and also very different. Not only did I put things into words, she said—which made for a degree of differentiation—but also she sensed that I had my own boundaries, that I didn't need her to be in perfect communion with me for my own purposes. Ms. I (chapter 9), who also showed pathology of boundary formation, addressed me formally by name several times in every session, thus working through the boundary issue in action. In each of these instances, it was my impression that the relational aspect of the encounter— the patient's sense of the analyst as a person with a sense of where his own boundaries lie—played an important role in the therapeutic gain, notwithstanding the extensive descriptive, interpretive, and reconstructive work that was also done via words.

And fourth, from the standpoint of the psychology of the ego, I will mention only some of the more general relational effects upon ego function that are inherent in the psychoanalytic encounter. I want to begin by referring, once again, to Loewald's (1960) paper, in which he addressed the function of speech as it works for the patient:

> Once the patient is able to speak, nondefensively, from the true level of regression which he has been helped to reach by analysis of defenses, he himself, by putting his experiences into words, begins to use language creatively, that is, begins to create insight. The patient, by speaking to the analyst, attempts to reach the analyst as a representative of higher stages of ego-reality organization, and thus may be said to create insight for himself in the process of language—communication with the analyst as such a representative. (p. 26)

The very act of putting experience into words, motivated as it is by the effort to "reach the analyst" and communicate gives form to (often) previously unformed experience and is part of a movement of such experience to higher levels of ego organization.

I would add that the analyst's silence is crucial here. The analyst's silence, and the patient's recumbent posture and free associative task not only create the conditions for a certain kind of *passivity* in the patient—wherein experience will flow, unscreened, sometimes regressively—but equally can be seen as creating the conditions for a certain kind of patient *activity*—giving shape to experience in the absence of any external shaping demands, putting things into words, and ultimately being both experiencer and observer of inner life.

I have made no attempt to be complete in describing potentially mutative effects of the relational aspect of the analytic encounter, but I have tried to show how the perspective of each of the four psychologies alerts us to aspects of those effects. They are largely inherent in the process; they do not require us to do anything special. They simply happen between people and, in analysis, they happen in ways that are functional (and malfunctional) in multiple ways for the patient. As the malfunctional, the pathological, uses of the relationship that the patient makes are pared away by interpretation, more functional uses of the relationship, serving growth, remain—often not noticed because largely conflict-free and not verbalized—though equally often recognized verbally between analyst and analysand as part of the total process.

In sum, then, I have tried in this chapter to conceptualize the mutative factors in psychoanalysis in a broad way. While interpretation in the transference can be most dramatic in its mutative potential, it is certainly not the whole of what takes place in an analysis. Overall I've suggested that, in the context of an intense and intimate relationship where things matter for the patient, both verbal interventions and relational factors have important mutative effects. I have used the four theories current on the psychoanalytic scene today as vehicles to explore the mutative potential of the psychoanalytic encounter. And I have tried to make two major points. The first is that interpretation (even interpretation in the transference, and well timed) has its major mutative potential when (to put it baldly and simplistically) it is right—that is, when it touches on something experientially (not necessarily consciously) valid in the patient—and to do that we have to interpret, varyingly, in the languages of each of the four psychologies—more in this one than that one for different patients, more of this one now and that one at another time in any single patient. And second the patient finds meanings in the relationship itself also along lines that we can conceptualize in terms of the four psychologies; this happens because processes active in patients (in each of these domains) find and recruit those meanings that work for inner life. When we are aware of and interpret those found meanings that are problematic in terms of the patient's pathology, when we pare them away, we still leave the patient with those found meanings that work for the patient in nonpathological ways, that foster change and renewed development.

Postscript

LOOKING BACK AT what I have written in this book, I am acutely aware that—although I have tried to stay close to the immediate phenomena of clinical work (and of development), and although I have given extensive illustrative clinical material—the final product still is only a pale approximation of the actualities of the psychoanalytic process. The mystery and creativity of that process, its long periods of uncertainty and its need for patience, its false turns, corrections, and sudden openings to major insight, can only be experienced, hardly conveyed. But I do believe that what I have presented here is nonetheless *some* approximation to that psychoanalytic process—perhaps just to the ways in which I currently do it—without the kinds of theoretical commitments that slant some published or presented case reports.

In concluding this book, I want to highlight a few points in the relation of a four psychologies conception to the process of clinical work.

First, I have found this perspective to be immensely freeing of the work. It

257

enables one to be respectful of and influenced by the writing of a wide range of contributors but, by focusing primarily on the *phenomena* they observed rather than the theoretical superstructures built on top of those, it mercifully deprives one of both the crutch and the entanglements of those superstructures. My position is hardly atheoretical, but it is (I hope) a theory that is close to phenomena: of the main lines of development, of psychological motivation and organization, and of the treatment process itself. It permits one to be eclectic in the clinical work exactly as much as one's patient is eclectic—that is, as much as the phenomena of the patient's intrapsychic life are describable and explainable in one set of terms and also in others.

Second, the analytic work does not consist principally of a set of interpretations or other interventions organized in relation to the phenomena of one or another of the four psychologies. The clinical illustrations that I gave in chapters 7 and 8 may seem to suggest this, but in them I reported instances in which material was *understood* in ways that could be subsumed within the terms of one or another or more of the psychologies. But much time in analysis involves redescribing and underlining what the patient is saying. This work goes on at such a low level of formulation (that is, so close to the reported phenomena themselves) that I find I cannot think of it in terms of the several psychologies. It is preparatory work, phenomena in search of a formulation. However, when things get understood, when the analyst can make sense of phenomena in some higher-order explanatory and linking way—at those times the understanding can and will be in the languages of one or more of the several psychologies—and in different ones at different times.

Third, I am often asked whether it is more difficult to work in this multimodel way, or I am simply told that it is too difficult. Isn't there too much to keep in mind? I am asked. I have several overlapping responses to this. One is that there is so much to keep in mind in an analysis anyway—so many potential meanings, even, say, just within the classical drive/structural theory—that adding more is like adding to infinity. But, from a contrary standpoint, there is nothing at all to keep in mind in an analysis except what the patient is saying; all the rest is clutter (until such point as theory helps clarification). And finally, whether or not it is difficult to keep so much in mind is not a relevant consideration; we have to keep in mind whatever will enhance the work. I maintain that a multimodel view does just that.

In fact I have gotten contrasting responses to the ideas described here when I have presented them earlier—from both experienced and relatively new clinicians. Many experienced clinicians have responded favorably to these ideas, saying that in fact they have come to work in such ways themselves and that it is good to see them formalized. Others, however—perhaps sometimes out of habit but certainly also out of successful experience in a particular way of working—have been unenthusiastic at best.

A parallel contrast exists in student and beginning clinicians as well. Some are uneasy, as though it all seems too complicated; they behave as if deprived of the crutch that a clear theory can give in the face of the therapeutic task which seems so overwhelming. Others, however, say, in effect, "What's all the fuss about?" As they told me when I began presenting these views, their training had familiarized them with drive, ego, object relations, and self theories. Whereas I was, intrapsychically, breaking away from the model in which I had been trained, they were hearing a way to use the many ideas to which they had been exposed and which were lying around waiting to be used. So they were comfortable with my formulation.

I hope that many of the readers of this book will have responded similarly.

References

Abraham, K. (1921). Contributions to the theory of the anal character. In *Selected Papers* (pp. 370–392). New York: Basic Books, 1953.

————. (1924). The influence of oral erotism on character formation. In *Selected Papers* (pp. 393–406). New York: Basic Books, 1953.

Alpert, A. (1959). Reversibility of pathological fixations associated with maternal deprivation in infancy. *Psychoanalytic Study of the Child, 14,* 169–185.

Bach, S. (1987). *Ego and self.* Paper presented at Third Annual Psychiatry Symposium of the Albert Einstein College of Medicine, New York.

Balint, M. (1968). *The basic fault.* London: Tavistock.

Bettelheim, B. (1943). Individual and mass behavior in extreme situations. *Journal of Abnormal Social Psychology, 38,* 417–452.

Blos, P. (1962). *On adolescence: A psychoanalytic interpretation.* New York: Free Press.

————. (1967). The second individuation process of adolescence. *Psychoanalytic Study of the Child, 22,* 162–186.

Bornstein, B. (1949). The analysis of a phobic child: Some problems of theory and technique in child analysis. *Psychoanalytic Study of the Child, 3/4,* 181–226.

Bowlby, J. (1969). *Attachment and loss: Vol. 1. Attachment.* New York: Basic Books.

―――. (1973). *Attachment and loss: Vol. 2. Separation: anxiety and anger.* New York: Basic Books.

―――. (1980). *Attachment and loss: Vol. 3. Sadness and depression.* New York: Basic Books.

Broucek, F. (1979). Efficacy in infancy. *International Journal of Psychoanalysis, 60,* 311–316.

Chethik, M. (1984). The "highly-functioning" borderline child: Some diagnostic thoughts and developmental considerations. Paper presented at meetings of American Psychoanalytic Association, New York.

Coen, S. J. (1986). The sense of defect. *Journal of the American Psychoanalytic Association, 34,* 47–67.

Cooper, A. M. (1987a). Changes in psychoanalytic ideas: Transference interpretation. *Journal of the American Psychoanalytic Association, 35,* 77–98.

―――. (1987b). Comments on Freud's "Analysis terminable and interminable." In *On Freud's analysis terminable and interminable,* ed. J. Sandler. *International Psychoanalytic Association Educational Monographs, 1,* 127–148.

Eissler, K. (1953). The effect of the structure of the ego on psychoanalytic technique. *Journal of the American Psychoanalytic Association, 1,* 104–143.

Ekstein, R., & Wallerstein, J. (1954). Observations on the psychology of borderline and psychotic children. *Psychoanalytic Study of the Child, 9,* 344–369.

Erikson, E. H. (1950). *Childhood and society.* New York: Norton.

―――. (1980). Plenary session discussion. First World Congress of Infant Psychiatry, Cascais, Portugal.

Escalona, S. (1963). Patterns of infantile experience and the developmental process. *Psychoanalytic Study of the Child, 18,* 197–244.

Fairbairn, W. R. D. (1941). A revised psychopathology of the psychoses and psychoneuroses. *International Journal of Psychoanalysis, 22,* 250–279.

Fleming, J. (1975). Some observations on object constancy in the psychoanalysis of adults. *Journal of the American Psychoanalytic Association, 23,* 743–759.

Fraiberg, S. (1969). Libidinal object constancy and mental representation. *Psychoanalytic Study of the Child, 24,* 9–47.

Freud, A. (1926). Introduction to the technique of the analysis of children. In *The psychoanalytical treatment of children* (pp. 3–52). New York: International Universities Press, 1946.

_____. (1936). The ego and the mechanisms of defense. In *The writings of Anna Freud* (Vol. 2). New York: International Universities Press, 1966.

_____. (1965). *Normality and pathology in childhood*. New York: International Universities Press.

_____. (1970). The symptomatology of childhood. *Psychoanalytic Study of the Child*, 25, 19–41.

_____. (1974). A psychoanalytic view of developmental psychopathology. In *The writings of Anna Freud* (Vol. 8, pp. 57–74). New York: International Universities Press, 1981.

Freud, S. (1897). *The origins of psychoanalysis* (Letter 69). New York: Basic Books, 1954.

_____. (1900). The interpretation of dreams. *The complete psychological works: Standard edition* (Vols. 4, 5). New York: Norton.

_____. (1905). Three essays on the theory of sexuality. *Standard edition* (Vol. 7, pp. 135–243).

_____. (1908). Character and anal eroticism. *Standard edition* (Vol. 9, pp. 169–175).

_____. (1911). Formulations on the two principles of mental functioning. *Standard edition* (Vol. 12, pp. 218–226).

_____. (1912). Recommendations to physicians practicing psychoanalysis. *Standard edition* (Vol. 12, pp. 111–120).

_____. (1914a). On the history of the psychoanalytic movement. *Standard edition* (Vol. 14, pp. 7–66).

_____. (1914b). Remembering, repeating, and working through. *Standard edition* (Vol. 12, pp. 147–156).

_____. (1915). Instincts and their vicissitudes. *Standard edition* (Vol. 14, pp. 117–140).

_____. (1916). Introductory lectures on psychoanalysis. *Standard edition* (Vol. 16, pp. 243–263).

_____. (1917). Mourning and melancholia. *Standard edition* (Vol. 14, pp. 243–258).

_____. (1919). Lines of advance in psychoanalytic therapy. *Standard edition* (Vol. 17, pp. 159–168).

_____. (1920a). Beyond the pleasure principle. *Standard edition* (Vol. 18, pp. 7–64).

_____. (1920b). The psychogenesis of a case of homosexuality in a woman. *Standard edition* (Vol. 18, pp. 147–172).

_____. (1923). The ego and the id. *Standard edition* (Vol. 19, pp. 12–66).

_____. (1926). Inhibitions, symptoms, and anxiety. *Standard edition* (Vol. 20, pp. 87–172).

————. (1930). Civilization and its discontents. *Standard edition* (Vol. 21, pp. 64–145).

————. (1933). New introductory lectures on psychoanalysis. *Standard edition* (Vol. 22, pp. 5–182).

————. (1937). Analysis terminable and interminable. *Standard edition* (Vol. 23, pp. 216–253).

Fromm-Reichmann, F. (1950). *Principles of intensive psychotherapy*. Chicago: University of Chicago Press.

Frost, R. (1971). The road not taken. In *Robert Frost's poems*, ed L. Untermeyer (p. 27). New York: Washington Square Press.

Gaensbauer, T. J. (1982). The differentiation of discrete affects: A case report. *Psychoanalytic Study of the Child*, 37, 29–66.

Goldberg, A. (Ed.). (1978). *The psychology of the self: A casebook*. New York: International Universities Press.

Greenacre, P. (1958). Toward an understanding of the physical nucleus of some defence reactions. *International Journal of Psychoanalysis*, 39, 1–8.

Greenberg, J. R., & Mitchell, S. A. (1983). *Object relations in psychoanalytic theory*. Cambridge, MA: Harvard University Press.

Greenson, R. (1967). *The technique and practice of psychoanalysis*. New York: International Universities Press.

Greenwald, A. G. (1980). The totalitarian ego: Fabrication and revision of personal history. *American Psychologist*, 35, 603–618.

Grunes, M. (1984). The therapeutic object relationship. *Psychoanalytic Review*, 71, 123–143.

Hartmann, H. (1939). *Ego psychology and the problem of adaptation*. New York: International Universities Press, 1958.

————. (1955). Notes on the theory of sublimation. *Psychoanalytic Study of the Child*, 10, 9–29.

Hegarty, A. (1989). Personal communication, New York.

Hendrick, I. (1942). Instinct and the ego during infancy. *Psychoanalytic Quarterly*, 11, 33–58.

Holt, R. R. (1972). Freud's mechanistic and humanistic images of man. *Psychoanalysis and Contemporary Science*, 1, 3–24.

————. (1976). Drive or wish? A reconsideration of the psychoanalytic theory of motivation. In *Psychology vs. metapsychology: Psychoanalytic essays in memory of G. S. Klein*, ed. M. M. Gill & P. S. Holzman. *Psychological Issues Monograph*, 36, 158–197.

Horner, T. M. (1985). The psychic life of the young infant: Review and critique of the psychoanalytic concepts of symbiosis and infantile omnipotence. *American Journal of Orthopsychiatry, 55,* 324–344.

Jacobson, J. G. (1983). The structural theory and the representational world. *Psychoanalytic Quarterly, 52,* 514–542.

_____. (1987). Personal communication.

Kanner, L. (1942). Autistic disturbances of affective contact. *Nervous Child, 2,* 217–250.

Katan, A. (1951). The role of "displacement" in agoraphobia. *International Journal of Psychoanalysis, 32,* 41–50.

_____. (1961). Some thoughts about the role of verbalization in early childhood. *Psychoanalytic Study of the Child, 16,* 184–188.

Kernberg, O. (1976). *Object relations theory and clinical psychoanalysis.* New York: Aronson.

Klein, G. S. (1976). *Psychoanalytic theory: An exploration of essentials.* New York: International Universities Press.

Klein, M. (1921–1945). *Contributions to psychoanalysis.* London: Hogarth, 1948.

Kohut, H. (1971). *The analysis of the self.* New York: International Universities Press.

_____. (1972). Thoughts on narcissism and narcissistic rage. *Psychoanalytic Study of the Child, 27,* 360–400.

_____. (1977). *The restoration of the self.* New York: International Universities Press.

Kris, E. (1955). Neutralization and sublimation: Notes on young children. *Psychoanalytic Study of the Child, 10,* 36–47.

_____. (1956a). The recovery of childhood memories in psychoanalysis. *Psychoanalytic Study of the Child, 11,* 54–88.

_____. (1956b). On some vicissitudes of insight in psychoanalysis. In *Selected Papers* (pp. 252–271). New Haven: Yale University Press, 1975.

Lichtenberg, J. (1983). *Psychoanalysis and infant research.* Hillsdale, N.J.: Analytic Press.

Loewald, H. W. (1960). On the therapeutic action of psychoanalysis. *International Journal of Psychoanalysis, 41,* 16–33.

_____. (1971a). On motivation and instinct theory. In *Papers on Psychoanalysis* (pp. 102–137). New Haven: Yale University Press, 1980.

_____. (1971b). Some considerations on repetition and repetition compulsion. *International Journal of Psychoanalysis, 52,* 59–66.

Lorenz, K. (1965). *Evolution and modification of behavior*. Chicago: University of Chicago Press.

————. (1970). *Studies in animal and human behavior* (Vol. 1). Cambridge, MA: Harvard University Press.

Madsen, K. B. (1959). *Theories of motivation: A comparative study of modern theories of motivation*. Copenhagen: Munksgaard.

Mahler, M. S. (1966). Notes on the development of basic moods: The depressive affect. In *Psychoanalysis: A general psychology*, ed. R. M. Loewenstein, L. M. Newman, M. Schur, and A. J. Solnit (pp. 152–168). New York: International Universities Press.

————. (1968). *On human symbiosis and the vicissitudes of individuation*. New York: International Universities Press.

————. (1972). On the first three subphases of the separation-individuation process. *International Journal of Psychoanalysis, 53*, 333–338.

————. (1975). On the current status of the infantile neurosis. *Journal of the American Psychoanalytic Association, 23*, 327–333.

Mahler, M. S., Pine, F., and Bergman, A. (1970). The mother's reaction to her toddler's drive for individuation. In *Parenthood: Its psychology and psychopathology*, ed. E.J. Anthony and T. Benedek. Boston: Little, Brown, 257–274.

————. (1975). *The psychological birth of the human infant*. New York: Basic Books.

McDevitt, J. B. (1975). Separation-individuation and object constancy. *Journal of the American Psychoanalytic Association, 23*, 713–742.

————. (1980). *Separation-individuation and aggression*. A. A. Brill Memorial Lecture, New York Psychoanalytic Society.

————. (1983). The emergence of hostile aggression and its defensive and adaptive modifications during the separation-individuation process. *Journal of the American Psychoanalytic Association, 31*, 273–300.

Mitchell, S. A. (1984). Object relations theories and the developmental tilt. *Contemporary Psychoanalysis, 20*, 473–499.

Modell, A. (1984). *Psychoanalysis in a new context*. New York: International Universities Press.

Noy, P. (1977). Metapsychology as a multimodel system. *International Review of Psychoanalysis, 4*, 1–12.

Osofsky, J. D. (Ed.). (1979). *Handbook of infant development*. New York: Wiley.

Parens, H. (1979). *The development of aggression in early childhood*. New York: Aronson.

Peterfreund, E. (1978). Some critical comments on psychoanalytic conceptualizations of infancy. *International Journal of Psychoanalysis, 59*, 427–441.

Piaget, J. (1937). *The construction of reality in the child.* New York: Basic Books, 1954.

———. (1952). *The origins of intelligence in children.* New York: International Universities Press.

Pine, F. (1970). On the structuralization of drive-defense relationships. *Psychoanalytic Quarterly, 39,* 17–37.

———. (1974). On the concept "borderline" in children. *Psychoanalytic Study of the Child, 29,* 341–368.

———. (1979a). On the expansion of the affect array: A developmental description. *Bulletin of the Menninger Clinic, 43,* 79–95.

———. (1979b). On the pathology of the separation-individuation process as manifested in later clinical work: An attempt at delineation. *International Journal of Psychoanalysis, 60,* 225–242.

———. (1981). In the beginning: Contributions to a psychoanalytic developmental psychology. *International Review of Psychoanalysis, 8,* 15–33.

———. (1982). The experience of self: Aspects of its formation, expansion, and vulnerability. *Psychoanalytic Study of the Child, 37,* 143–167.

———. (1984). The interpretive moment. *Bulletin of the Menninger Clinic, 48,* 54–71.

———. (1985). *Developmental theory and clinical process.* New Haven: Yale University Press.

———. (1986a). On the development of the "borderline-child-to-be." *American Journal of Orthopsychiatry, 56,* 450–457.

———. (1986b). The "symbiotic phase" in the light of current infancy research. *Bulletin of the Menninger Clinic, 50,* 564–569.

———. (1988). The four psychologies of psychoanalysis and their place in clinical work. *Journal of the American Psychoanalytic Association, 36,* 571–596.

———. (1989). Motivation, personality organization and the four psychologies of psychoanalysis. *Journal of the American Psychoanalytic Association, 37,* 27–60.

———. (in press). The place of object loss in normal development. In *The problem of loss and mourning: psychoanalytic perspectives,* ed. D. R. Dietrich and P. Shabad. New York: International Universities Press.

Rapaport, D. (1951). Toward a theory of thinking. In *Organization and pathology of thought,* ed. D. Rapaport (pp. 689–730). New York: Columbia University Press.

———. (1953). Some metapsychological considerations regarding activity and passivity. In *The collected papers of David Rapaport,* ed. M. M. Gill (pp. 530–568). New York: Basic Books, 1967.

————. (1957). The theory of ego autonomy: A generalization. In *The Collected Papers of David Rapaport*, ed. M. M. Gill (pp. 722–744). New York: Basic Books, 1967.

————. (1960a). On the psychoanalytic theory of motivation. In *Nebraska Symposium on Motivation*, ed. M. R. Jones (pp. 173–247). Lincoln: University of Nebraska Press.

————. (1960b). The structure of psychoanalytic theory. *Psychological Issues Monograph, 6.*

Rapaport, D., and Gill, M. M. (1959). The points of view and assumptions of metapsychology. *International Journal of Psychoanalysis, 40,* 153–162.

Redl, F. (1951). Ego disturbances. In *Childhood Psychopathology*, ed. S. I. Harrison and J. F. McDermott (pp. 532–539). New York: International Universities Press, 1972.

Rosenfeld, S. K., and Sprince, M. P. (1963). An attempt to formulate the meaning of the concept "borderline." *Psychoanalytic Study of the Child, 18,* 603–635.

Sander, L. W. (1977). Regulation of exchange in the infant-caretaker system: A viewpoint on the ontogeny of "structures." In *Communicative structures and psychic structures*, ed. N. Freedman and S. Grand (pp. 13–34). New York: Plenum Press.

Sandler, J. (1960). The background of safety. *International Journal of Psychoanalysis, 41,* 352–356.

————. (1976). Countertransference and role responsiveness. *International Review of Psychoanalysis, 3,* 43–47.

————. (1981). Unconscious wishes and human relationships. *Contemporary Psychoanalysis, 17,* 180–196.

Sandler, J., and Rosenblatt, B. (1962). The concept of the representational world. *Psychoanalytic Study of the Child, 17,* 128–145.

Sandler, J., and Sandler, A.-M. (1978). On the development of object relationships and affects. *International Journal of Psychoanalysis, 59,* 285–296.

Schafer, R. (1983). *The analytic attitude.* New York: Basic Books.

————. (1986). Personal communication. New York.

Schulman, G. (1988). Personal communication, Helsinki.

Segel, N. P. (1981). Narcissism and adaptation to indignity. *International Journal of Psychoanalysis, 62,* 465–476.

Settlage, C. F. (1977). The psychoanalytic understanding of borderline and narcissistic personality disorders: Advances in developmental theory. *Journal of the American Psychoanalytic Association, 25,* 805–833.

Singer, M. (1988). Fantasy or structural defect? The borderline dilemma as viewed from analysis of an experience of nonhumanness. *Journal of the American Psychoanalytic Association, 36,* 31–60.

Southwood, H. M. (1973). The origin of self-awareness and ego behavior. *International Journal of Psychoanalysis, 54,* 235–240.

Spence, D. P. (1982). *Narrative truth and historical truth: Meaning and interpretation in psychoanalysis.* New York: Norton.

Spiegel, L. A. (1959). The self, the sense of self, and perception. *Psychoanalytic Study of the Child, 14,* 81–109.

Spitz, R. A. (1957). *No and yes.* New York: International Universities Press.

Stern, D. N. (1985). *The interpersonal world of the infant: A view from psychoanalysis and developmental psychology.* New York: Basic Books.

Stoller, R. J. (1968). *Sex and gender.* New York: Science House.

Stone, L. (1954). The widening scope of indications for psychoanalysis. *Journal of the American Psychoanalytic Association, 2,* 567–594.

————. (1986). Personal communication.

Stone, L. J., Smith, H. T., and Murphy, L. B. (1973). *The competent infant: Research and commentary.* New York: Basic Books.

Strachey, J. (1934). The nature of the therapeutic action of psychoanalysis. *International Journal of Psychoanalysis, 15,* 127–159.

Sullivan, H. S. (1953). *The interpersonal theory of psychiatry.* New York: Norton.

Waelder, R. (1936). The principle of multiple function: Observations on overdetermination. *Psychoanalytic Quarterly, 5,* 45–62.

Weil, A. (1953). Certain severe disturbances of ego development in childhood. *Psychoanalytic Study of the Child, 8,* 271–287.

————. (1956). Certain evidences of deviational development in infancy and early childhood. *Psychoanalytic Study of the Child, 11,* 292–299.

Werman, D. S. (1984). *The practice of supportive psychotherapy.* New York: Brunner/Mazel.

White, R. W. (1959). Motivation reconsidered: The concept of competence. *Psychological Review, 66,* 297–333.

————. (1963). Ego and reality in psychoanalytic theory: A proposal regarding independent ego energies. *Psychological Issues Monograph, 11.*

Winnicott, D. W. (1956). Primary maternal preoccupation. In *Collected Papers* (pp. 300–305). New York: Basic Books, 1958.

————. (1958a). The capacity to be alone. In *The maturational processes and the facilitating environment* (pp. 29–36). New York: International Universities Press, 1965.

————. (1958b). *Collected Papers*. New York: Basic Books.

————. (1960a). Ego distortion in terms of true and false self. In *The maturational processes and the facilitating environment* (pp. 140–152). New York: International Universities Press, 1965.

————. (1960b). The theory of the parent-infant relationship. In *The maturational processes and the facilitating environment* (pp. 37–55). New York: International Universities Press, 1965.

————. (1963a). The development of the capacity for concern. In *The maturational processes and the facilitating environment* (pp. 73–82). New York: International Universities Press, 1965.

————. (1963b). Psychiatric disorders in terms of infantile maturational processes. In *The maturational processes and the facilitating environment* (pp. 230–241). New York: International Universities Press, 1965.

————. (1965). *The maturational processes and the facilitating environment*. New York: International Universities Press.

————. (1967). Mirror-role of mother and family in child development. In *The predicament of the family*, ed. P. Lomas. London: Hogarth Press.

Wolff, P. H. (1959). Observations on newborn infants. *Psychosomatic Medicine*, *21*, 110–118.

Youngerman, J. K. (1979). The syntax of silence: Electively mute therapy. *International Review of Psychoanalysis*, *6*, 283–295.

Index

271

Listening, psychoanalytic; neutrality, 8, 19, 50–54; phrasing, 42; question asking, 8, 44; and resistance, 50–51; tact and timing, 8, 42, 126, 230; and transference, 50–51, 248; verbal interventions, 248–51
Thumbsucking, 9–11, 29, 31, 188
Toilet training, 109, 186, 243
Transference, 14, 18, 19, 124, 255; and clinical techniques, 50–51, 248; and drives, 45; in Freud, 36; narcissistic, 30, 253–54; neurosis, 25, 30; oedipal, 193; repetition in, 26
Trauma, 45, 48, 126, 171–72; and ego defects, 201, 207; strain, 81–82, 96, 196
Trust, 65, 66; and ego defects, 200, 202–3; vs. mistrust, 74–75, 103

Urges, 4, 10, 13, 23; biological, experienced as internal, 10; and cognition, 91; lasting, power of, 28, 33; psychic representation of, 10, 33, 90–91, 96, 145; Winnicott on, 10; see also Drive(s)

Verbal interventions, 248–51
Verbalization, 53, 87, 109, 229, 250–51, 254–55; see also Speech

Waelder, Robert, 80, 88
Wallerstein, Judith, 113
White, Robert, 67, 78
Will, 66, 151, 180
Winnicott, Donald W., 53, 104, 244, 252; environmental provision, 61; "going on being" in, 9–10, 31, 63; "holding" aspect of analytic situation in, 52; and object relations theory, 29; self in, concept of, 15, 38, 66, 161, 234
Wishes, 13, 60, 95; development of, 63; and fantasies, 33; focus on, in psychoanalysis, 29–30; and object relations, in early childhood, 35; for repetition, of gratifying experiences, 14–15; sexually powered, 6, 252; see also Drive(s)
Wolff, Peter, 9, 236

Youngerman, Joseph, 201